GAINING WEIGHT?

HIGH FRUCTOSE CORN SYRUP AND OBESITY

Dee Takemoto, Ph.D. and
Joanne McIntyre, R.D.C.S.

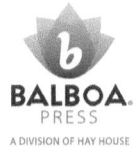

BALBOA.
PRESS
A DIVISION OF HAY HOUSE

Balboa Press books may be ordered through booksellers or by contacting:
Balboa Press
A Division of Hay House
1663 Liberty Drive
Bloomington, IN 47403
www.balboapress.com
1-(877) 407-4847

ISBN: 978-1-4525-4359-8 (sc)
ISBN: 978-1-4525-4361-1 (hc)
ISBN: 978-1-4525-4360-4 (e)

Library of Congress Control Number: 2011963456

Printed in the United States of America

Balboa Press rev. date: 01/25/2012

Introduction

So, you have been trying to lose weight! Well, join the 70 per cent of Americans who are overweight, already exercise, and really do not eat that much. What's the problem? The problem is the toxic foods you are eating, not the calories. Things like artificial sweeteners, high fructose corn syrup, and leached toxins from plastic are messing with your metabolism and appetite centers. You gain weight no matter what you do. This book will show you why we are poisoning ourselves and how to stop. And, in the process, we will show you how to lose weight easily, getting rid of that unwanted tummy fat.

The authors wish to thank the many scientists who have dedicated their lives to understanding the metabolic effects of what we eat. We have only cited a few of their works herein. We apologize if you are not included but know that without your work our people would not be as healthy.

Contents

140 IS THE NEW 110 –

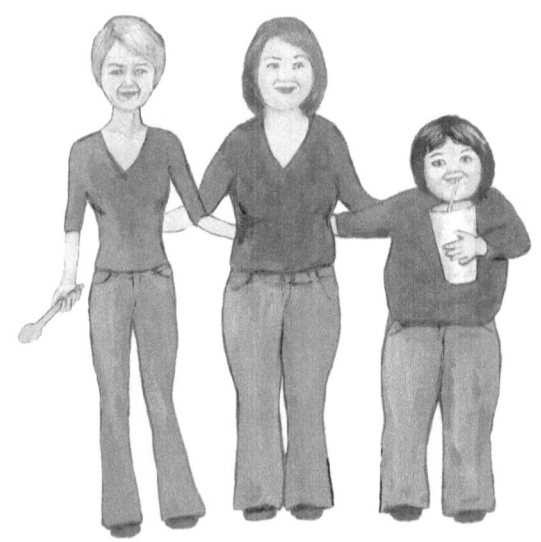

"GAINING WEIGHT?"

Last summer my sister and I were painting in my studio in the backyard, commenting on this and that. We got around to health issues since she has been teaching in that area, to college students, for about 32 years. Both of us always struggle to keep our weight down, and, had been discussing the trend in weight gains among students. She told me about her students who had lost weight by just giving up high fructose corn syrup. Thus, the idea for this book was hatched. I begin with a story about my son.

Last year, my son had been searching a popular free dating website and was growing discouraged by the fact that prospects were worse in the smaller city where he was now living. My husband suggested to him that he just let me take over, for him, on the site. To our surprise he agreed. Being his mother, of course I looked at all the best looking women who said all the right things. I was thinking about having beautiful grandchildren and being able to get along well with my future daughter-in-law. I was also worried about the fact that he was looking a lot at women from outside of his geographic area, because he could find women that were more girlish looking for their ages. I didn't want him to drive too far, after all, I am his mom.

The few women that he had dated previously were hard to talk to because they weren't accustomed to our family habit of sarcastic humor. They did appear, however, to be slimmer and more feminine than the group of women listed on the website as living nearer to him.

I've struggled to maintain a normal weight all my life, due to some social and family pressure, of course, but probably mostly due to the fact that, growing up in southern California in the 1960's, the men all wanted a woman who weighed less than 120 pounds. There were so many fat jokes among the men that we were afraid to gain a single pound. Those same men could grow a huge beer gut and feel they were still "Mr. Macho". But we couldn't.

If a young woman ever wanted to sample all the holiday treats, she would have to diet the week before or the week after the party to make sure her husband or boyfriend wouldn't be able to say anything about the obvious three pounds that she had gained. I remember my older sister fasting for four or five days before Thanksgiving so that she could eat anything that she wanted. The problem with that approach is that, when you fast like that, your stomach gets used to it and, when you try to eat a lot, you fill up too fast. And, you get full even before the dessert comes!

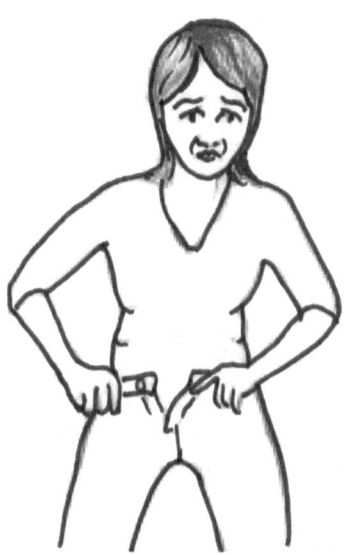

Even after having three children, I was expected to stay thin. I remember a couple of times that I gained five pounds over the holidays and thought that my favorite pants had gotten shrunk in the dryer. I couldn't get the button hole over to the button and was appalled at the little mounds of fat between the two sides of my jeans zipper. Looking back at my old photos, when my friends and I were in our mid 30's, and had two or three children, I can see that we all looked like we weighed around 115 lbs. But most of us still felt fat and we were trying to get down to that ever elusive 110.

So, for my son, I was looking for a female, 30 to 40 years old who was, in the terms used on the website, "thin or athletic". To my surprise, all the athletic women appeared, in their pictures, to be overweight. The weirdest part, to me, was that the obese women, (according to the body mass index chart), thought that they were only a few pounds overweight, and, those that looked overweight classified themselves as average. And, the athletic girls looked, at least to my son, like they had better go to the gym two more times a week.

Since I know how easy it is to gain weight when you get pregnant, (yes, I was thinking of grandchildren) I wanted my future daughter-in-law to be a normal weight to begin with.

So, at that point, being a determined mom, I decided to do an advanced search. This time I specified "thin." I was amazed to see that, with a couple of other specifications, such as a "nonsmoker" and someone between 5 foot and 5 foot 8 inches tall, the search, within a 10 mile area, came up with <u>zero</u>. I broadened the search to 25 miles, then to 50, and then to 100, and finally came up with two ladies. Los Angeles was within that 100 mile area! What happened to us?

In the next few weeks, I started looking around at the beach where my husband and I take walks on the weekends. This was southern California; mind you, land of the "stars". All those beautiful bodies have disappeared from the beaches! Once, I saw a group of teenagers celebrating one of their coming of age parties for 15 year old girls. They were all posing and getting their pictures taken, in their formal attire, out on the rock jetty in Oceanside. The girls were all in strapless gowns and the boys where in new white shirts and black dress pants. All of the girls and boys were overweight or obese!

The enormity of the problem hit me! I thought this was only a problem in places like the south, where I went to visit my daughter and her children. This was a state where the natives ate things like "hush puppies" and corn chowder and sausage gravy on biscuits. Yummy, but you might as well rub it on my hips!

Once, on a visit there, with my husband, we were in a large retail store and my husband spotted a whole rack full of pants that were about six feet around the waist and were just labeled as XL. He thought it was a joke. I assured him that there were people that large. But, not so many, in the recent past!

Now the obesity problem is everywhere. It's an epidemic! No longer could my son insist on dating a thin woman. There weren't any available! Why?

Vanity Sizing

If you are over 55 you may remember something that I brought to my sister's attention a short time ago. We used to wear bigger sizes. Right now I am almost the exact size in weight and measurements that I was 40 years ago but I remember distinctly that the dress I bought for my older sister's wedding was a size 8. Now I wear a size 4. My sister was dubious at first when I told her this. I used to sew my own clothes when I was a stay at home mom, so I decided to try to find some old dress patterns from the 60's. When I sent her some old patterns I found, she was dumbfounded. She responded, "Wow! The difference is amazing, 5 to 10 inches. The hip size for a size 12 was 34" on one pattern. Now, on the recent standard for sizing in the US on the chart below you can see that the hip size for a size 12 is 41".

On the patterns I found for sale on-line, a dress size of size 12 had a bust size of 32 inches, a waist size of 25 inches, and a hip size of 34 inches. No wonder they always said that Marilyn Monroe was a perfect size 12.

Now you can be 7 inches larger in the hips and still say you wear size 12. The waist size of 25" in the sizes 10 and 12 in the patterns I found are now for a size 2.

You can check out lots of vintage patterns for sale on eBay and many other web sites. They give you the sizes and the measurements for each size.

Sample Of Sizing In The 60s

UK	8	10	12	14	16
USA	6	8	10	12	14
CONTINENTAL	36	38	40	42	44

JAPANESE	7	9	11	13	15
BUST	32in	34in	36in	38in	40in
WAIST	24in	26in	28in	30in	32in
HIP	35in	37in	39in	41in	43

A few weeks ago my husband and I were sitting in the yard and a couple we knew walked by and decided to sit down with us and talk. She told me that she recently went to buy some jeans and was having a hard time getting jeans that fit right. She ended up getting some that were the same size as the ones she wore when she was in college. She thought, "This can't be right. I know I'm 30 pounds heavier than I was then!"

See the recent jeans size chart below. The garment industry is just trying to get you to buy clothes and ignore how big you're getting. I used to be a size 8 in the 60's. Now all my jeans are a size 4. By this chart, it appears that Australian sizing is the closest to what ours used to be.

JEANS SIZES

US	US	UK	FRANCE	GERMANY	ITALY	AUSTRAILIA
XXS	0	2	32	30	34	4
XS	2	4	34	32	38	6
XS/S	4	6	36	34	38	8
S	6	8	38	36	40	10
M	8	10	40	38	42	12
M	10	12	42	40	44	14
L	12	14	44	42	46	16
L/XL	14	16	46	44	48	18
XL/1X	16	18	48	46	50	20
1X/2X	18	20	50	48	52	22
2X	20	22	52	50	54	24
3X	22	24	54	52	56	26
3X	24	26	56	54	58	28

KIDS TOO?

After having worked in the pediatric medical field for many years, I have recently begun to notice that there are also a lot more overweight children. When I was a kid there were usually only one or two overweight children in a class of 30 kids. Unfortunately most of the other kids made fun of them and the nice kids would whisper that they must have a "thyroid condition". Now, this is a phenomenon I never thought I'd see in my lifetime. What are their parents allowing the children to eat?

Most of the kids came into the clinic between breakfast and lunch, and, they were carrying a package of chips and a boxed fruit-flavored drink with a straw. By eleven o'clock, they were promised fast food meals, if they behaved. So, why were they so hungry all the time even though they never stopped eating?

Were they eating breakfast?

I asked the kids what they had for breakfast, and, most of them had already eaten cereal, toast, and/or donuts. I know that, if I only eat something sweet in the morning, I am hungry again, in a couple of hours. But, I never remember being allowed, when I was younger, to eat in the doctor's office. It must be what the parents were giving their children for breakfast. Even though the food was full of calories, it was not satisfying them. They were still hungry! This book will tell you why. Parents all seem to believe that a whole baby bottle full of fruit juice is appropriate for a one-year-old. Are doctors telling parents to do this? And, what was in that fruit juice?

Maybe I go a lot on intuition, but, I always figured that, if it doesn't come like that, in nature, you shouldn't consume it that way. It takes about four good sized oranges to make a large glass of fresh squeezed orange juice. You only need one whole orange with the fiber around each wedge to feel perfectly satisfied that you have had enough orange juice. The rest in that bottle has just too many calories, and, as we are about to explain, <u>too much high fructose corn syrup (6 grams of fructose in an orange *vs* 10 grams in the juice)</u>.

Can you imagine how many apples it took to make that baby bottle full of apple juice so devoid of fiber that it has no resemblance to apples? Did you know it is probably full of high fructose corn syrup?

It has only been in the past few decades that there is even a home device for extracting juice out of things like carrots and apples. I had a friend who used to use two pounds of carrots in her juicer each morning for her glass of carrot juice. Her grocery bill was phenomenal. And, by the way, she weighed close to 300 pounds. So drinking carrot juice was not going to help her lose weight.

Once, a couple brought their 15 year-old son to the Cardiologist whom I was working with. They complained that their son was short of breath. He weighed 400 pounds! These parents seemed clueless of this fact. I felt like asking them if they would get short of breath if they had to carry around two 100 pound bags of cement all day. The poor kid probably didn't even want to get out of bed in the morning. He had to have been obese at a very early age. When did we get oblivious to obesity? When did it become OK for a 15 year old to weigh 400 pounds?

Whose fault was it? Obviously his parents didn't plan this.

Our society has learned to accept obesity at a great cost to health. It is now OK for our kids to be overweight or obese at even a young age. I recently went to a popular animation movie where even the main character, a ten year old boy, was overweight. The cartoonist had actually drawn the character to be obese. This was obviously an attempt to reach out to what had become the normal child viewing audience. It is now acceptable in our society to have kids who are overweight. Considering the metabolism of a kid, can you imagine how much messed up food it must take to create an obese child?

"Food" Additives

I used to read every label on canned or packaged foods that I ate, looking for unnecessary salt, sugar, preservatives, coloring, and lists of things that didn't sound like food. We will show you how to do this. I bet you have not done this and that is one of the problems. We have lost our ability to read labels and tell what we are eating.

One of the things I noticed, in the seventies, was that a lot of food began to have "corn sweeteners" listed on those labels. I just figured that they were trying to make everything taste better. At the time, I was trying to avoid sugar, and I figured corn syrup was just as bad as sugar. We will describe, in this book, that it is actually worse than sugar! I looked for the can of beans with the ingredients that mom used to make "homemade beans" with; beans, salt, onions, maybe a little bacon, and, some celery. When fruit was out of season, I'd looked for the can of peaches that said "in its own juice". I figured that, if the fruit was ripe, it wouldn't need sugar. I actually found applesauce made with nothing but apples! This is really hard to find now. Most cans of fruit now contain high fructose corn syrup. And, we are just too busy anymore to read those labels and see what has high fructose corn syrup. We will give you a list, in the Appendix, of foods without this unhealthy food additive.

Canned fruit used to come with "sugar" when I was a kid. Now it almost always contains high fructose corn syrup. I figured that they had added the "high fructose" phrase to make people think it was somehow from fruit fructose. But you should not be fooled. Even though fruit has fructose it's also loaded with fiber, and, not high fructose corn syrup. This fact alone, we will show you, has contributed to the growing trend in obesity in this country and, maybe, in your family.

I remember having an old bottle of corn syrup in the cupboard. Occasionally some recipe in my cook book would call for it. The bottle would sit there for years and, in a pinch, if I ran out of pancake syrup I could use it for less tasty syrup on my pancakes. Now, you drink it every day, as a sweetener in soft drinks. And, your kid's breakfast cereal is filled with it.

As I checked labels, I started seeing "corn syrup" not only in beans, but, also in vegetables and just about every packaged food that used to contain sugar, and, sometimes even in odd things like catsup. I thought maybe there was a really big surplus of corn in our country. I wasn't too political at the time, being kind of a hippie artist housewife, in the hills of northern California, but I had read that they were subsidizing farmers not to grow certain crops and that imports of certain foods were being limited.

One of these was sugar which had been replaced by high fructose corn syrup! Lobbying power, anyone?

In the coming chapters we will show you how bad your diet has become, and, what you are allowing to happen to yourself and your children. By not being aware that you are consuming an unnatural diet, filled with high fructose corn syrup, you are gaining weight younger, and, at a higher rate than ever before, in human history! And, we will show you how this leads to a dangerous condition called Metabolic Syndrome, even in your kids!

We will give you a list of brand name foods that do not contain high fructose corn syrup. You will come to know that, unlike what those ads tell you, high fructose corn syrup is not the same as sucrose and, yes, your body does know the difference. By substituting these food brands into your diet you will be on the way to increased health.

We hope that this book will help you and your family to get back on track to a healthy life.

And to start you on the right track, let's begin with reading labels.

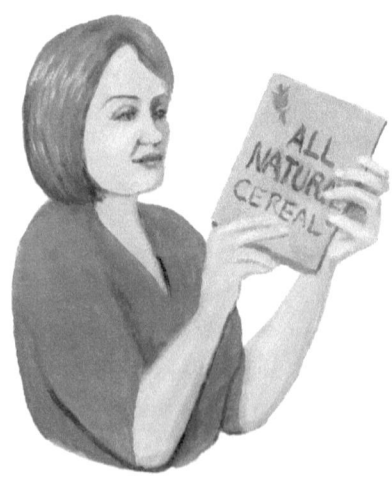

READ THE LABEL!

was probably in my teens when I first started reading labels. I was a teen bride and pregnant at sixteen. My older sister (18 years old) and I got married within a week of each other and our daughters were born within two months of each other. By my eighth month I had gained 35 pounds and the doctor told me my blood pressure was up. High blood pressure runs in the family. He wanted me on a salt-free diet. I know that some of you have had to do this and it is not easy. It takes a long time to adjust to a low salt diet. Things taste better with salt!

In this chapter, we will tell you how to read labels, and, we start with the basics, salt.

SALT

Sodium chloride, brine, sea salt; no matter how you name it, there have been whole cities, countries, and cultures built around salt. Entire countries have perished in wars over salt. The use of salt to preserve food allowed armies to travel by foot or in boats to take over other countries and change the geopolitical structure and our history. In Roman times, their armies took over cities and countries just because they had salt. People were sold into slavery to work in salt mines and were said to be worth their weight in salt. Salt can be used to pickle, preserve, change the taste, prevent bacterial growth, and take the water out of foods. We would not have developed as a culture without salt. However, too much salt is not a good thing.

The Food and Drug Administration recommends no more than 2400 milligrams (mg) of salt per day. Our salt is chemically something called sodium chloride, one atom of sodium and one of chlorine. Since there is natural sodium in things like meat and fish and celery, going on a salt-free diet was, for me, an effort in order to keep my sodium intake down to about 1000 milligrams per day.

My husband was overseas with the Navy when I was pregnant and I was staying with my parents. Mom helped me by buying me salt-free bread and salt-free butter. What a treat that was! If it were not for the grape jelly, it would have tasted like greasy cotton. After a month or so of reading every label to look for salt and for any food that tasted ok without it, I was surprised at how my taste buds seemed to adjust over time. Scrambled eggs with only pepper actually started tasting good. Fresh ocean fish tasted salty with no salt added. Actually, I could taste things that I formerly thought had very little taste without salt. My body had adjusted back to normal. Nevertheless, remember, it takes a while for this to happen so if you want to lower your salt, do it slowly over about 3 months. Just start by salting something about half as much.

After giving birth and being able to resume my old diet, I was appalled at how salty potato chips and onion dip and pickles tasted. For some reason most canned soup has more salt than you need for the whole day. If you are on a low sodium diet look at the labels and beware. I discovered that a fast food hamburger with the three little slices of dill pickle contained my entire daily requirement of sodium (salt). Forget the fries, for multiple reasons that you can read about elsewhere. By the way, if your ankles swell up, you are probably taking in too much sodium. This can make your blood pressure go up.

The sodium in that salt has to be pumped right out of each of your cells because the amount of sodium in a cell has to remain so much lower than what the level is outside of each cell. This is so that all those metabolic reactions can take place. Remember that salt "pickles" things and the same thing would happen to the insides of your cells. Unfortunately, pumping out all that sodium that you eat takes energy, and, at first, your cells try to dilute it by taking in water. Then, your ankles swell. Over time, your blood system gets damaged and your blood pressure goes up.

Your heart uses sodium as an ion, a charged atom used to generate an electrical current. However, your heart only needs a little of it. If it gets flooded with sodium, it has to work overtime to get rid of it. So, heart problems can also result from too much salt.

Below is a chart with a few common foods with their sodium (salt) contents. You will find, as you read labels, that salt has been added to almost everything. Of course, if you add more salt or catsup to anything it is even higher.

Sodium in select common foods

FOOD	WEIGHT (G)	PORTION	SODIUM
mg Burrito/ beans and meat	115.5	1 burrito	668
Cheeseburger, single meat patty	102	1 sandwich	500
Cheeseburger, large single with vegetables	219	1 sandwich	1108
Cheeseburger, large with bacon	195	1 sandwich	1043
Cheeseburger, regular, double patty	155	1 sandwich	636
Hamburger, large single meat patty	218	1 sandwich	824
Submarine sandwich with roast beef	216	6 inch	845
Fish sandwich/ sauce and cheese	183	1 sandwich	949
Roast beef sandwich, plain	139	1 sandwich	792
Chicken fillet sandwich, plain	182	1 sandwich	957

FOOD	WEIGHT (G)	PORTION	SODIUM
Chicken, breaded and fried, boneless	106	6 pieces	513
Croissant with egg cheese and bacon	129	1 croissant	889
English muffin/ egg cheese & bacon	137	1 muffin	729
Hot dog	98	1 sandwich	670
Nachos and cheese	113	6-8 nachos	816
Pancake with butter and syrup	232	2 pancakes	1104
Pizza/cheese, meat and vegetables	79	1 slice	789
French fries	85	1 small	168
French fries	169	1 large	335
Taco salad	198	1 1/2	762

Sodium in Meat and Poultry

FOOD	WEIGHT (G)	PORTION	SODIUM
Beef stew, canned	232	1 cup	937
Beef, cured dried beef	28.35	1 oz.	984
Beef, ground, extra lean, broiled	85	3 oz.	60
Bologna, beef and pork	56.7	2 slices	578
Chicken pot pie, frozen	217	1 small pie	857
Chicken breast, meat only, broiled	86	½ breast	64
Chicken drumstick, meat only, broiled	44	1 drumstick	42
Chicken hot dog, meat only	45	1 hot dog	617
Beef hot dog, meat only	45	1 hot dog	462
Ham, sliced, extra lean	56	2 slices	800
Lamb, lean, broiled or baked	5	3 oz.	71
Pasta with meat balls and tomato sauce	252	1 cup	1053
Pork sausage, fresh cooked	26	2 links	336
Pork sausage, fresh cooked	26	1 patty	350
Salami, cooked, beef or pork	57	2 slices	605
Turkey, roasted	84	3 oz.	66

Sodium Content of Fish and Seafood

FOOD	WEIGHT (G)	PORTION	SODIUM
Catfish, raw	85	3 oz	51
Clam, raw	85	3 oz	48
Cod, Atlantic, canned	85	3 oz	185
Crab, Alaskan King	85	3 oz	715
Lobster, cooked	85	3 oz	320
Lobster, raw	85	3 oz	180
Haddock, cooked	85	3 oz	75
Oyster, raw	85	6 medium	177
Salmon, canned	85	3 oz	471
Salmon, fresh cooked	85	3 oz	56
Sardines	85	3 oz	430
Shrimp, canned	85	3 oz	144
Swordfish, raw	85	3 oz	46
Trout, brook, raw	85	3 oz	40
Trout, rainbow, raw	85	3 oz	70
Tuna, albacore, raw	85	3 oz	34
Tuna, white, canned in water	85	3 oz	320

CARBS, AND, I LOVE DESSERT!

Later in my twenties, while trying to lose that last twenty pounds, after having two babies, I looked at labels for their calorie content. I discovered that fat has twice as many calories, gram for gram, as carbohydrates. I tried high carbohydrate diets, low fats diets, and just about everything in between. I tried the T-factor diet, the Atkins diet, the Weightwatchers diet, a diet with only grapefruit and hard-boiled eggs, a high protein diet, diet milk shakes, and whatever was that year's latest fad.

I never seemed to be able to stay on any one diet for more than a few weeks but they all encouraged me to exercise, which, by the way, only made me hungrier.

Of course, all of the diets advise you not to have sweets, which I love. I found that most packaged sweets have a ridiculous amount of calories. Check the labels! Since I could not lose weight without limiting myself to about 1500 calories per day, I thought it would be foolish to waste it all on a 350 calorie candy bar. If I did fall under its spell, it seemed like I was hungrier than if I had never had it. Of course, I'm finding out now that if the candy had sugar instead of high fructose corn syrup like it used to when I was a kid, the little bit of sugar may have held me over till the next meal.

Once I lost 10 pounds in one week by eating only chewable protein tablets with a rare low calorie meal. I would always gain a little back after I got off a diet. Overall, I found that if you cut out the most useless calories, fats (cheese is bad) and sugars (pass up that donut shop), you will lose weight over time.

After about 3 years, I got back down to my ideal weight, which, for me, is when you can see light between my thighs. I do not think I could have done it, though, if I had not learned to read labels. I learned that some foods have so many calories that they should probably be eliminated from the human diet, for instance, cream. Also, look at the label on most non-dairy coffee creamers. I know people who put three of those in one cup of coffee. Most of it is full of high fructose corn syrup, and a bunch of unreadable "stuff". But, if you have to add something to your coffee just add one teaspoon of regular table sugar (sucrose).

The FDA only allows something to be called "sugar" if it is sucrose from sugar cane or beets. The corn refining industry has applied to the FDA to be able to call high fructose corn syrup "corn sugar". I think this would be very confusing since, chemically, it is not sucrose but free fructose and free glucose.

The best diet, in my opinion, is one that makes you feel good (not psychologically for the moment, i.e. chocolate), does not make you hungry all the time, and helps you to look good (i.e. no zits and good fits). What works for me are some lean protein and a lot of vegetables. But, try getting your kids to go for that! I don't want to eat that <u>only</u> either. There go all the usual snacks and desserts. And, I love dessert!

Mom made dessert for every evening meal. Before we were finished eating, the question from everyone was "what's for dessert?" We would save room for whatever it was. Sometimes it was something light, like Jell-O with bananas. Not much room required, so eat another piece of bread or, when we got it, put some whipped cream on top of the Jell-O. What I really loved was cake with powdered sugar icing, made with Crisco, the preferred baking grease of the day. She made this great recipe, chocolate mayonnaise cake, so moist with chocolate icing, and all that grease. Yum! All of her desserts were homemade and most of it was full of sugar and fat, but still, all of us were thin. When I was thirteen, I remember being so thin that I wore two slips under my straight skirt so my hip bones wouldn't protrude.

And, our drink of choice from my earliest memories was a popular powdered drink mix, each quart made with about a cup of sugar. But, there were five of us and Mom only made one 32 ounce container. We only had it at mealtime, not all day long, whenever we wanted it. We could also choose milk with our meal and that goes a lot better with cake any way. I'm not saying that we didn't have cavities in our teeth, but we were still thin.

Now, I do not recommend that anyone eat dessert on an everyday basis because most of us do not make homemade desserts. If you do love desserts like me, you should make sure they contain a natural sweetener and not <u>high fructose corn syrup</u>. And never use those artificial sweeteners for your kids.

The following recipes present three choices for making brownies. The first one shows the ingredients in a well-known box mix. Notice that it contains high fructose corn syrup as well as a preservative (potassium sorbate, prevents molds and fungus from growing) and something called *xanthan gum.*

Xanthan gum is used to thicken foods but is made from wheat and corn so beware if you have food allergies! It is also a powerful laxative. I found that out the hard way when I tried to substitute no fat half-in-half in my coffee. Too bad they can't find some kind of thickener with that same luscious texture but without the laxative effect. In addition, if you'll notice, the oil in recipe #1 is partially hydrogenated (some hydrogen is added to make it a more saturated fat) which we now know could cause you to have bad cholesterol (LDL) if in a trans form. The niacin, thiamin, riboflavin, and folic acids are all B vitamins and are not bad for you. Soy lecithin means a fat from soybeans. Of course, we have no way of knowing what "artificial and natural flavors" means.

The second one is an ingredient label from an off-brand brownie mix, which I actually purchased because it has no high fructose corn syrup, and, because my husband loves brownies. It is probably not much better, but at least it doesn't appear to have any preservatives or the high fructose corn syrup. It does contain guar gum, a thickener from the guar bean, also a laxative. (Note: If you get diarrhea immediately after eating at a salad bar, ask the servers if they put an anti-bacterial spray on their foods. It is also a strong laxative.)

The last recipe lists the ingredients out of my mother's cookbook. As you can see, it uses just ordinary food ingredients that you can buy at the grocery store. This is your best choice. Of course, you are better off with only one or two of mom's brownies if you are trying to lose weight. I have not listed the calories or fat content in any of these recipes. That information is always listed under "Nutritional Content" which is different from the ingredients. One more thing; the ingredients are listed by amount in the food, with the highest level of ingredients listed first. So, in recipe #1 the biggest ingredient is sugar.

INGREDIENTS – RECIPE 1

> Sugar, Enriched Flour Bleached (Wheat Flour, Niacin, Iron, Thiamin Mononitrate, Folic Acid), Chocolate Chunks (Sugar, Chocolate Liquor, Cocoa Butter, Soy Lecithin, Vanillin), Chocolate Flavored Syrup (Sugar, Water, High Fructose Corn Syrup, Cocoa Processed With Alkali, Salt, Citric Acid, Potassium Sorbate (Preservative) Xanthan Gum, Artificial and Natural Flavor),Partially Hydrogenated Vegetable Oil (Soybean and Cottonseed Oil).

Citric acid adds tartness so you have a better appetite and eat more brownies. It is not the same as vitamin C, which is ascorbic acid. Ascorbic acid or vitamin C is a great anti-oxidant. If taken in chewable form it can help with those scratchy, itchy eyes on a high pollen day, can help get rid of zits, and helps prevents colds.

Notice the salt also added to almost everything. You will see that in good old fashion home recipes too. This adds a little flavor and helps prevent bacterial growth. But, only use a pinch!

INGREDIENTS – RECIPE #2

> INGREDIENTS: SUGAR, ENRICHED BLEACHED FLOUR (BLEACHED WHEAT FLOUR, MALTED BARLEY FLOUR, NIACIN, REDUCED IRON, THIAMINE MONONITRATE, RIBOFLAVIN, FOLIC ACID), PARTIALLY HYDROGENATED SOYBEAN AND COTTONSEED OILS, COCOA, DICALCIUM PHOSPPHATE, CORN STARCH,

DEXTROSE, SALT, FOOD STARCH, DEXTROSE, SALT, FOOD STARCH-MODIFIED, NATURAL AND ARTEFICIAL FLAVORS, GUAR GUM, AND NONFAT DRY MILK. **CONTAINS WHEAT, SOYBEAN AND MILK.**

INGREDIENTS – RECIPE 3

Cake Brownies

1 ¼ cups sugar, ¾ cups butter, ½ cup unsweetened cocoa powder, 2 eggs, 1 teaspoon vanilla, 1 ½ cups all-purpose flour, 1 teaspoon baking powder, ¼ teaspoon baking soda, 1 cup milk

EATING FOR HEALTH

When I was in my thirties I stopped drinking caffeine, in either coffee or tea, for a few years because I was starting to get a lot of sore lumpy places in my breasts and the doctor said it was aggravated by caffeine. I noticed that a lot of sweet stuff that I regularly ate tasted much better with a cup of coffee. Donuts and sweet rolls did not go well with herbal tea. Half of the experience was lost.

Since I would often embarrass myself at church functions by returning to the sweet roll table, again and again, I decided to discipline myself by cutting out sugar. Wow, was that a major decision. I started looking at labels again. Sugar was everywhere! That was when I really started noticing that they were starting to substitute high fructose corn syrup for the sugar in almost everything, from peanut butter to beans. The list of ingredients in some of those food packages was so long, and, I did not even understand why half of it was in there. Cellulose Gum? (A thickening ingredient made from a plant). I had to start going to health food stores to get fresh ground peanuts and oatmeal instead of granola.

At first, eliminating sugar was so difficult that I had to occasionally drink unsweetened apple juice or eat really sweet fruit or I would have terrible cravings. Sometimes I would resort to a teaspoon of sugar in my tea. Well, OK, more than sometimes. But, after a while I noticed the same effects as when I was on the salt-free diet. In a few months, that apple juice with high fructose corn syrup tasted disgustingly sweet and, so, I switched to the juice without those added sweeteners. Then, later I found myself watering the drink down because it was also too sweet. As with salt, my body had adjusted to accept high sugar and very sweet foods. My metabolism had adjusted. It took about three months to adjust it back to normal. So if you do decide to give up salt or some sugar be sure to take your time and do it slowly over 3-4 months. Otherwise, the food will taste terrible to you and you won't stick to it.

I found out that I would have to cut out things like catsup and barbeque sauce and pickle relish and numerous other things that were sweetened with sugar or corn syrup. They do make varieties without sweeteners or just a little sugar. Meanwhile I noticed, while checking the labels, that most of these condiments had switched to high fructose corn syrup when they had formerly used sugar when I was a kid. And, things tasted even sweeter.

Before I stopped eating sugar, I had also noticed that when I had eaten my favorite boxed cereal or processed sweets for breakfast in the morning that I would be hungry again in less than two hours. I always thought that it was because I had not eaten enough protein, even though I had it with milk I remembered having cereal in the morning when I was a kid and being able to wait until noon for the lunch bell to ring. Could it be the high fructose corn syrup? Yes! I had eaten the stuff but it did not get into my appetite center to say, "full now". Cereals have changed in the last 30 years so that, with the use of high fructose corn syrup, your kids are always hungry.

This was the other reason I tried to fix my eating habits, besides losing weight. It was to try to fix my health problems. We will talk about some serious problems known as Metabolic Syndrome later.

Z<small>ITS</small>

When I was around the age of eleven, I began to be prone to getting pimples on my face. I hated this. Once, a snooty girl at school asked me, "why don't you do something about your skin?" At the sensitive age of eleven I was very humiliated. I had no clue what to do about it besides the few topical ointments sold over the counter and I was already trying that. I was told it had something to do with hormones because it happened more at certain times of the month. It did not do any good to just wash my hair more or use "hypoallergenic" make-up.

When I was in my twenties and even thirties, I was still occasionally getting big zits on my chin or right in the middle of my cheek. I noticed that if I had peanut butter and jelly sandwiches three days in a row, I would always get a big sore one no matter what time of the month it was. I was really conscious of dietary fat at the time because of so much dieting, so I figured it was the fat in the peanuts that, if you read the label, is appreciable. It could have been that I had sensitivity to peanuts, which is common. Whatever it was, I found that if I avoided peanut butter I rarely had skin problems.

Even in my forties and fifties, I could bring one on by eating too much peanut butter. And, by then I was using the kind with only peanuts and salt because, by then, I was an avid label reader. I know not everyone gets zits from peanut butter. My sister gets them from potato chips, even the all-natural ones. So sometimes, it may be one of those weird "food additives". The point is you have to pay attention to what you eat. Sometimes you can avoid zits by not eating a particular brand of cookies, like my daughter. If you are allergic to a food and it gives you zits the next day then you have to substitute a different brand. No amount of face chemicals will make those zits disappear because you are eating foods that you are allergic to. You have to switch brands.

Below are the ingredient lists from two peanut butter labels. You can see that I have not given it up altogether since I have the labels. The one with the corn syrup is actually a "low fat" peanut butter. In other words, low fat does not mean less calories or less high fructose corn syrup. The second one has only peanuts and salt but includes an apology for having used equipment that had other ingredients on it.

Note: magnesium oxide, ferric orthophosphate, and copper sulfate are sources of magnesium, iron, and copper, respectively. Fully hydrogenated vegetable oil means saturated fat and mono- and diglycerides also means fat.

PEANUT BUTTER #1

> INGREDIENTS: PEANUTS, CORN SYRUP SOLIDS, SUGAR AND SOY PROTEIN, CONTAINS LESS THAN 2 PERCENT HYDROGENATED VEGETABLE OILS (GRAPESEED AND SOYBEAN), SALT MONO AND DIGLYCERIDES, MOLASSES, PERIDOXINE HYDROCHLORIDE, MAGNESIUM OXIDE, ZINC OXIDE, FERRIC, FERRIC ORTHPHOSPHATE, AND COPPERSULPHATE.

I always thought that zinc oxide was used in deodorants, rubber cement and diaper rash ointment The one below sounds safer.

PEANUT BUTTER #2

> INGREDIENTS: DRY ROASTED PEANUTS, SALT. MADE ON EQUIPMENT SHARED WITH TREE NUTS. FACILITY PROCESSES WHEAT, MILK, EGG, AND SOY. NO PRESERVATIVES

BEWARE OF BLUE FOOD!

In the seventies when my son was around 6 years old I took him to the doctor because he was having trouble focusing in school. From all the descriptions of his shenanigans, the doctor deducted that he had ADHD. He said that he could put him on some drug or I could try the new popular diet that was out. He must have seen me coming because I was not about to put my son on drugs. How many doctors suggest altered diets now?

He referred me to a book about food additives and artificial coloring that Dr. Feingold had written (The Feingold Diet). I got the book and started eliminating all the additives he recommended including preservatives, food dyes and monosodium glutamate, a common flavor enhancer, which is also a neurotransmitter and can cause migraine headaches.

At the time, a commercial fruit punch that was bright red was the main drink served to children at parties and in the church and commercial care centers. The Food and Drug Administration now has a site to look up the dyes. The initials FD&C before the color stands for "Food, Drug and Cosmetics" and the number is the FDA code for the structure. Some have been known to be carcinogenic (cause cancer). One has caused deaths. (http://www.fda.gov/ForIndustry/ColorAdditives/ColorAdditivesinSpecificProducts/InMedicalDevices/ucm142395.htm).

If the dye is called a "Lake", it means that it does not dissolve in oil but does stay around longer. You will see both Lakes and FD&C numbered dyes in many types of foods. The FDA only started to regulate them in the last 20 years or so. There are some natural colorings for foods. When we make soap in the lab part of my course, I have the students use paprika or lemon oil for orange or yellow coloring. Annatto, from the bean, is used for a natural red color. But, beware of blue food. There are very few natural things that are blue except maybe those poisonous frogs in South America.

The red dye in the fruit punch drink was considered one of the biggest offenders on the Feingold Diet. Do a search on red food dyes and you will never want to buy colored candy for your kids again. Next to the red dye, for terrible effects, was yellow dye. I suddenly made a strong correlation in my mind because my son used to be the calmest baby and toddler until I started taking him to day care centers. The neighbor where he sometimes played served a red colored drink to her kids constantly. I started following the diet for him and within 3 weeks, I could not believe he was the same kid. I think we are doing the same thing to our kids now with those colored little boxed juice drinks. And, diagnosed ADHD is on the rise.

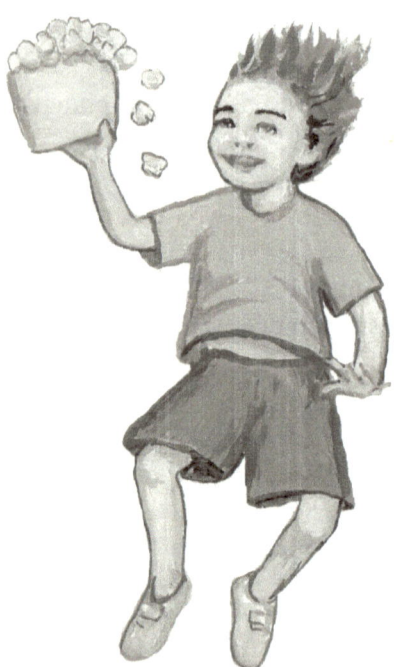

Once, after I had followed all the recommendations for a couple of months, my family went out together. We were watching a game from some bleachers at a school. My son was fine until someone gave him a bag of bright yellow popcorn. Within twenty minutes, he became totally uncontrollable, running into people and climbing on all the railings. To me this was proof that the dye had something to do with it. This diet had me looking at every label and reading everything about the kinds of foods that have a stimulating effect on the brain such as, believe it or not, raisins and anything with monosodium glutamate in it (most canned soups).

The Feingold Diet has remained controversial since the 1970's but I totally believe in it and so does my now grown up son. There seems to be a resurgence of interest in it because several years ago I tried to look it up and found very little. Now it is easy to find on the internet. I recommend it to parents with hyperactive children, especially to those whose kids are already on ADHD drugs and who act like zombies with no personality. You can check it out on Feingold.org or on Wikipedia. I believe that you should first check your child's food before ever putting them on one of those strong neuro-active drugs.

The main thing that I have learned from all of these everyday problems is that you have to start reading the labels. I've been told that you should never go into the middle aisles of the grocery store; just stay on the outside edges where the fresh produce, meat, dairy products and breads are. Then you will avoid a lot of preservatives and colors. That is not entirely true. Much of the processed lunchmeats are on the outside and contain nitrates, high salt, high fructose corn syrup and many other things that are not healthy. If you do venture into those forbidden aisles, please, for your health and for your children's health, read the labels.

Here are a couple of ingredient labels which contain food dyes. The first one is for barbeque-flavored potato chips. The second one is for an orange colored puffy cheese snack, which, if I eat one, I have a hard time stopping. They also give me zits.

INGREDIENTS FOR BARBEQUE-FLAVORED POTATO CHIPS

Ingredients: Potatoes, Sunflower Oil And/ or Corn Oil, Authentic BBQ Seasoning (Less Than 2% Of The Following: Sugar, Corn

Maltodextrin, Dextrose, Brown Sugar, Onion Powder, Monosodium Glutamate, Spices, Salt, Tomato Powder, Molasses Solids, Autolyzed Yeast Extract, Modified Corn Starch, Artificial Color [Including Yellow 5 Lake, Yellow 6 Lake, Blue 2 Lake, Red 40, Yellow 5, Blue 1], Sunflower Oil, Garlic Powder, Corn Starch, Citric Acid, Natural And Artificial Flavors, Natural Mesquite Smoke Flavor, Disodium Inosinate, Disodium Guanylate), And Salt

For your information, the Disodium Inosinate and Disodium Guanylate are added in place of Monosodium Glutamate so that they can sometimes say, "no MSG". Don't be fooled, they have a similar effect, although this particular product has all three. Another note, do you ever wonder how they get "natural mesquite smoke flavor? What, do they burn it over a mesquite fire?

INGREDIENTS FOR CHEESESNACKS

Enriched corn meal (corn meal, ferrous sulfate, niacin, thiamin mononitrate, riboflavin, and folic acid), vegetable oil (contains one or more of the following: corn, soybean, or sunflower oil), salt, maltodextrin, sugar, monosodium glutamate, autolyzed yeast extract, citric acid, artificial color (including red 40 lake, yellow 6 lake, yellow 6, yellow 5), corn syrup solids, partially hydrogenated soybean and cottonseed oil, hydrolyzed soy protein, cheddar cheese (cultured milk, salt, enzymes), whey, onion powder, whey protein concentrate, corn syrup solids, natural flavor, buttermilk solids, garlic powder, disodium phosphate, sodium diacetate, sodium caseinate, lactic acid, disodium inosinate,

disodium guanylate, nonfat milk solids, sodium citrate, and carrageenan.

Oh, and how about some food dye for your baby?

STRAWBERRY READY TO FEED (FOR BABY BOTTLES)

Water, Dextrose. Less than 2% of the Following: Citric Acid, Potassium Citrate, Sodium Chloride, Sodium Citrate, Natural Flavor, Sucralose, Acesulfame Potassium, Zinc Gluconate, <u>FD&C Red #40, and FD&C Blue #1.</u>

OK, so let's go over the ones that we've missed so far. Lactic acid gives things a sour flavor, sodium diacetate is for that vinegar flavor, and disodium phosphate is to keep things dry. That leaves carrageenan, something you will see in a lot of processed foods such as soft ice cream. It is from seaweed and gives things that gel texture. It is what makes toothpaste look like that.

WHAT IS CHEESE-FOOD?

I was recently called for a phone interview with a student who was a member of the University Newspaper staff. He was asking about a controversy related to a fast food taco place. They were being investigated for not having all beef in their "all beef" tacos. The student was surprised that something advertised as "all beef" only had to be a certain percent beef. As it turned out the fast food place had gone to a lowered beef content and substituted beef with oatmeal. I told the student that it was certainly not all beef but that oatmeal was, at least, not unhealthy. I also told him that there were Food and Drug Administration rules about the percent's of foods required to label something as "all-beef" or "all-cheese" , but, that it could usually be from many parts of that cow. For a fast food place to sell a meat sandwich it must be about 40% meat. But, the labels can be very misleading.

For example, there is a famous fast food place, which advertises roast beef sandwiches. Their roast beef is not from the "roast" section of the cow, but is all beef, from the tongue.

Cheese is famous for having many names and varieties including "processed cheese", "cheese slices", "prepared cheese", and, my favorite, "cheese food". You even have a spreadable version and one that can be squeezed from a bottle. American cheese is one form of processed cheese, which also contains, in addition to the cheese, emulsifiers, extra salt, food dyes, and whey, an extract from cream. "Cheese food" has to have at least 51% cheese. Pasteurized process cheese spread can be between 44-60% cheese.

This brings me to a last point, brand foods do differ from one country to another. Canada and Europe generally do not add high fructose corn syrup or corn syrup to most of their products, even if it is the same thing. Here are two examples, copied from the labels of Cheese Spread from Canada and the USA.

Canadian Cheese Spread

Modified milk ingredients, cheese (modified milk ingredients, bacterial culture, salt, calcium chloride, color, rennet (a cheese culture agent), and or microbial enzymes), water, maltodextrin, sodium phosphates, salt, sodium alginate, ground mustard, spice, color, sorbic acid, lactic acid

USA Cheese Spread

Whey, canola oil, milk protein concentrate, maltodextrin (a food additive to make thing more solid), sodium phosphate, contains less than 2% of whey protein concentrate, salt, lactic acid, sodium alginate, mustard flour, Worcestershire sauce (vinegar, molasses,

corn syrup, water, salt, caramel color, garlic powder, sugar, spices, tamarind, natural flavor), sorbic acid as a preservative, milk fat, cheese culture, oleoresin paprika, (color), annatto (color), natural flavor, enzymes.

Don't get me wrong. I am not knocking cheese you can squirt from a bottle. It makes a good cheese sauce or dip. But, if it is from the USA it does have a little corn syrup and a bunch of other stuff.

RAMEN NOODLES

OK, I had to include a separate section on Ramen noodles because that is the staple of my students. For one part of my college class, I have them take a food and write out the label, and, what each item was. I have included that in the Appendix section. After class one student, an exchange student from Japan, told me that she only ate Japanese food at home and that she made it by herself so could not find anything with the required 15-20 ingredients in it. I asked her if she ate Ramen noodles. She told me "Yes" but she also fixed that for herself from the package. I told her to use that as a label. I have given the ingredients for a brand of packaged Ramen noodles with beef broth below. T-BHQ, tertiary butyl hydroquinone, is a preservative commonly used in foods that sit on the shelf for a long time. Sodium and potassium carbonate are used to keep the pH acidic. Foods that are more acidic perk up your appetite so you eat more.

BOXED INSTANT SOUP MIX

Noodle: enriched flour, wheat flour, iron, thiamine, riboflavin, folic acid, vegetable oil, salt, sodium tripolyphosphate (used in detergents), potassium carbonate, sodium carbonate, sodium alginate (a thickening

agent), chili, paprika, tocopherol (vitamin E), T-BHQ

Soup Base: salt, hydrolyzed soy, corn, and wheat protein, monosodium glutamate, soy sauce powder, maltodextrin, chili and other spices, caramel color, autolyzed yeast extract, onion powder, garlic powder, dehydrated cilantro, beef powder, beef fat, disodium guanylate, disodium inosinate, dehydrated leeks, hydrolyzed wheat gluten, sugar.

It would be much better, I told my student, if you just used the noodles, very little of the stock, then added your own fresh foods. But, her diet was much better than that of some of my students. After handing in their 3 day dietary diaries (see the Appendix), the most common diet was cereal, Ramen noodles, pizza and beer, and, almost nothing fresh, or what I call "live food".

MY FOOD COMES IN PLASTIC

At the end of this chapter, I want to discuss, not your food, but what it is wrapped in. I know that plastic has been in the news a lot lately and that most of you know that something with the initials, BPA, is toxic and can be found in your food. So what is it? BPA, or bisphenol A, is a component of all plastics. That would include your plastic water bottles, food wrapping, plastic baby bottles, toys, and plastic milk cartons. It comes in various varieties because producers of plastic bottles can use up to 20 different types of chemicals to make one single baby bottle.

The Environmental Protection Agency (EPA) has a label code for the types of plastic, which looks like the picture below. Each triangle has a number inside and this determines what the primary type of plastic is. For example, #3 stands for PVC, polyvinyl chloride, a packing plastic, while #2 means HDPE, high-density polyethylene, for milk bottles and other liquid containers.

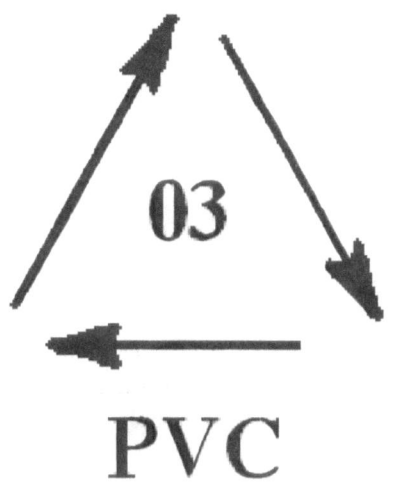

PVC

The BPA in plastic was not thought to be a problem until about 2 years ago when blood tests were done on adult volunteers and then on infants. We were all loaded with toxic plastic substances.

After that time the EPA and the plastic agencies made versions of bottles which were advertised as BPA-free. Everyone read about it, bought the newer and safer bottles, and thought that they had solved the problem. But, those nasty research articles kept coming out linking BPA in neonates, newborns, and infants to the increase in ADHD, autism and many other developmental and mental disorders.

The EPA then did another study to determine the levels of leaching out of the chemicals from bottles after washing with water, alcohol, or a combination, after heating, microwaving and exposure to the sunlight. They reported that you should not even leave the BPA-free bottles in the sunlight, and, that new toys, pacifiers, and flame-retardant-coated clothes for babies would release BPA into the environment and continued to show up in infant's blood. (ehponline.org). The article can be found on Pubmed and the first author is Chun Z. Yang, doi:10.1289/ehp.1003220, available at http://dx.doi.org. The authors did an exhaustive study to determine the relationship between BPA leaching from bottles and something else just as dangerous.

It had been suggested from several studies in humans that BPA caused elevated estrogen levels in men, women and infants. This is especially bad because estrogen causes developmental defects in fetuses, damage to children, and obesity in adults. The study tested all known plastic using water and alcohol washes, heat and sunlight, and microwaving. They found that the estrogenic activity was not linked to the BPA and that all plastics, no matter what they advertised, had the estrogenic activity. This included the special, all natural organic brands and the ones advertised as BPA-free. And, baby bottles were exceptionally bad.

This means that the known increase in ADHD and autism could very well be linked to the toxic exposure of our children at a very young age and even before they are born. The authors went on to suggest that it was the actual heat process of making the plastic that does this and that more work needs to be done to develop ways to make plastics which are safe for foods. But, for now, they are not. So, you do have to read those labels too!

A code label on the bottom of your plastic could look like this:

Resin identification code for PET

It's kind of hard to read on some small bottles. I had to use a magnifying glass on one. You can look up the latest research and dangers of each type and make your own educated decision on how you can limit the use of any of these products.

One product, <u>high fructose corn syrup</u>, is bad enough to take an entire chapter.

DOES YOUR BODY KNOW THE DIFFERENCE?

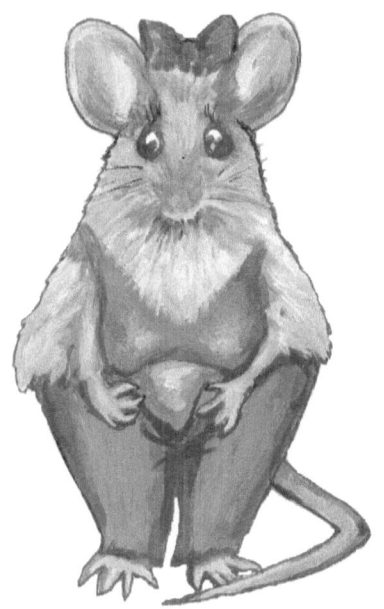

HFCS vs Sucrose (Table Sugar)

Does your body know the difference? You've seen the commercials on TV, put out by the High Fructose Corn Syrup (HFCS) refining industries, those funny ones, where someone questions another on why they are concerned about HFCS consumption. The "friend" says, "It's natural, all sugar and your body doesn't know the difference". First let's hit that last comment. Take a look at the chemical structures drawn below. I know, they are strange and look like maybe connected chicken wire with O's and H's hanging off of them. The one on the left is really only a tiny bit different from the one on the right. Check out the left side with the O= and the one on the right with the –OH instead. The left one also has a CH_3 stuck on that the one on the right does not have. So what are they? Well, the one on the left is Testosterone and the one on the right is Estradiol (estrogen). Yes, one is for boys and one is for girls. Only that tiny difference! YOUR BODY KNOWS THE DIFFERENCE! I always start my class lecture at the beginning of the semester with this slide. It serves to tell them how the human body can spot only slight differences in chemical structures. I have taught this and other Biochemistry courses to college students for 32 years. It is only recently, due to alarming increases in students' weight, that I have also gone on to explain what HFCS does.

Testosterone   Estradiol

Now take a look at the chemical pictures below. What kind of differences do you see there? The one on the right is a bigger "thing" and has a bigger ring. The one on the left has a smaller ring and CH_2OH hanging off at two places, top left and bottom right The one on the left is fructose and the one on the right is glucose. Does your body know the difference? Yes! When you say you have low blood sugar you are talking about glucose which is 99.99% of the sugar in blood. When you talk about sugar for brain food or energy you are talking about glucose since the brain only uses glucose for energy (unless you are starving then it can also use something called ketone bodies).

Fructose   Glucose

I then invite my students to take a test. I ask them to agree to eat only foods without HFCS in them for the remainder of the semester. I tell them not to cut calories or any of their favorite foods or even "diet". They just have to substitute those foods without the HFCS in them. This is hard without the Table in the Appendix. Several of my summer students patiently went through the grocery store, line by line, and read all the labels. You have learned how to read labels in the previous chapter. It is getting easier now that some suppliers and brands have changed and labeled their products, "no high fructose corn syrup". Some producers were just lucky and never had HFCS in their foods anyway. They didn't have to change anything. Other companies have volunteered to do this after reading the scientific studies. But I tell my students to read the labels anyway, just to be sure. Weight loss, for those who agree to the challenge has been from about 14 to 21 pounds, That is in a single semester, or four months, at my University. Not bad for only leaving out one thing. In general these were students who did not exercise too much and were definitely not the Division 1 athletes in the course. None of them complained about feeling hungry because it was not a diet. It was just a no HFCS regime.

Now, I am sure that you could lose more weight faster if you did more exercise and ate less. But, if you are reading this book, you probably have already tried everything else. Let's face it, those other diets made you hungry or you craved weird foods, or you had to buy pre-packaged up-scale versions of frozen TV dinners. Awful, and, you probably gave up on those diets after 3-6 months. This "diet' really is not a diet at all. It gets at one major source of the huge weight gain in our population. One that has contributed to obesity in kids as young as 5, and, has caused at least a 20% increase in high blood pressure, a 35% increase in type 2 diabetes, and a 30-60 per cent increase in overweight or obese people in the U.S. in the last 30 years. This is called Metabolic Syndrome and we will go over that in a separate chapter. Moreover, this perfectly correlates with the increase in sugar consumption, almost entirely through an increase in the consumption of; you got it, high fructose corn syrup! (Note to my readers; you can find all of these statistics on the CDC page on obesity). I want you to become pro-active so check out that page now at www.cdc.gov.

The fact is, you have evolved to use glucose as your primary sugar source in what we biochemists call "Central Metabolism". Central Metabolism means the common end point for what you eat. If you eat meat it gets broken down to amino acids, then, changes inside cells to a final carbon source called acetyl CoA, which is linked to the production of what we biochemists call the "money" of the cell, ATP. Central Metabolism does this. If you eat fats, these fats still get changed into things that go into Central Metabolism at some point along the pathway, to acetyl CoA and ATP. And, the initial thing that Central Metabolism starts with is glucose, not fructose. Fructose gets into Central Metabolism another way and that's the problem. It makes fat! And that is what is making you fat even though you exercise and diet. Glucose does not do this. It is the natural start point for Central Metabolism, and the normal sugar in the body. Don't misunderstand me, if you consume too many calories you will gain weight. Everyone knows this. But, HFCS makes the situation even worse. We will describe how this happens, in this chapter.

Diabetics use a color method to measure their blood sugar. They are measuring glucose. Yes, fructose is classified as a sugar, and, yes it can be changed to glucose using a bunch of different enzymes in your body. But, YOUR BODY KNOWS THE DIFFERENCE. You have pathways in all your cells for breaking down food, to nutrients, then, to molecules which will eventually enter what we call Central Metabolism. So what do you think the starting point for Central Metabolism is? You got it, glucose! But you don't use glucose in your cakes or fudge because, in taste tests, it's just not sweet enough for you. You can check out the degree of sweetness for the sugars by looking for fructose on Wikipedia. They list something called a "sweetness factor" which means a taste test. Glucose gets 74.3, sucrose gets 100, and fructose gets 173, or about 2.3 times sweeter than glucose. No wonder they use it. Taste tests probably showed a preference for it since you and I love sweets. Those taste tests were what made Coca Cola and Pepsi switch to HFCS (and lower cost)[2]. Pepsi introduced a version with sucrose, Pepsi Throwback. Coca Cola has not followed suit and you would have to get glass bottles of Coca Cola made in Mexico to get a version without HFCS. Coke Classic is not the original recipe, as it also contains HFCS.

We mostly use granulated sugar in our coffee, something called table sugar, and, chemically called sucrose. This is shown below. Yes, it is made from one fructose and one glucose (50:50) stuck together (called a chemical bond) in equal amounts. But, HFCS is not the same. It is an altered form of starch with a final product of free glucose by itself and free fructose by itself, not stuck together. If it contains more than that, for fructose, it's called high fructose, and, if it comes from corn syrup that would be called high fructose corn syrup (HFCS).

Ah, you ask, but so what, how would my body know the more or less part? It's only 5% more fructose than what you have in table sugar (sucrose), right? Kind of like asking if 0.02% blood alcohol is the same as 0.08%. Well, the highway patrol knows that difference and over the long haul so does your body, when ingesting that extra fructose! And, HFCS has a different kind of fructose. It is not connected to glucose like it is in table sugar. It is a single, unattached fructose, called "free fructose". Not free, as in no cost. As we will see, free fructose has a great cost, to your health and can result in Metabolic Syndrome.

As an example of the slight differences in concentrations of things in your body, normal blood glucose levels are from 3.6 – 5.8 millimolar (abbreviated mM) while a diabetic has around 5 – 7 mM blood glucose. That's also <u>not</u> a big difference in numbers. But, one person is normal and the other has a life threatening disease (diabetes).

High-fructose corn syrup is called glucose-fructose in the UK and glucose/fructose syrup in Canada [1-3]. In this country, the one used in soft drinks is HFCS 55 (55% fructose and, about 45% glucose). There is also HFCS 45 and even HFCS 90 (only used as a blender)[4-6]. When you read the labels, something we have shown you how to do in the previous chapter, you will see HFCS called that, or, corn syrup, or fructose corn syrup. They are all the same thing. Recently, the Corn Refiners' Association has requested permission to label HFCS as "corn sugar". This occurred on September 14, 2010[7]. We find this even more confusing to you. Since sugar is not sugar, is not sugar, wouldn't it be better to label it as, say, HFCS55 or HFCS45 or whatever it really is? But anyway, where does this stuff come from? Well, not from natural foods.

WHERE DOES THE STUFF COME FROM?

First, let's be straight, the Food and Drug Administration has stated that HFCS is safe for consumption so you are not eating something toxic like mercury. But, while cane sugar and beet sugar are mostly pure sucrose, HFCS is a combination of single glucoses, single fructoses and some sucrose. In other words table sugar does not have fructose by itself since it is stuck onto glucose when it gets into your body. HFCS has some free fructose all by itself. It depends on which type of HFCS is used. Honey is similar to HFCS but has many other components from those bees, like proteins. And besides, we don't consume large quantities of it so it's not an issue for your waist-line. In contrast, during the last 30 years HFCS consumption has increased enormously in the U.S. In 1970 the average person consumed about 0.5 pounds per year of HFCS. By 2000 that number jumped to 42 pounds per year. Last year, that jumped to about 60 pounds per year. At the same time, sucrose consumption went from around 70 pounds per year in 1970 to 40 in 2010[8]. Much of the increase in HFCS consumption is from soft drinks. As we will discuss below, fructose is not used in the body in the same way as sucrose or glucose. YOUR BODY KNOWS THE DIFFERENCE!

So how is HFCS made? Corn is the starting point, and, I don't want to bad mouth corn because it is a very good source of carbohydrates and proteins in the diet. Native Americans ate it long before we did and they did just fine, thank you very much. And, contrary to what some may think, the corn farmers do have other very good uses for their corn, like animal feed for those great steaks, and as a bio-ethanol source. In fact only about 5% of the U.S. corn goes to HFCS. It's really the corn refining industry that is putting out those ads. Maybe the industry would be better off taking some of that ad money and funding research into exactly what per cent of fructose is OK (doesn't cause you to have a big tummy). This is similar to the history of trans fats. Do you remember that margarine used to have trans fats in it? The industry got busy and found out how to make their product without it so that your cholesterol would not get elevated.

So anyway, back to where it comes from. Corn is harvested and milled (ground) into meal to eventually get corn starch, the stuff you put into gravy to make it thicker. Starch, also called pectin when making jelly, is actually all glucose connected in long chains, together. The only difference between starch and pectin and the form stored in your muscles, glycogen, (what runners do when they "carb-load", increase muscle glycogen) are the numbers of those branched connections called alpha-1,6. Those make branches while the alpha 1,4 make long chains. So corn starch is all glucose and not a problem with causing obesity.

You can keep using it to thicken foods and sauces without fear. But it is not sweet because glucose in long chains does not taste sweet[9].

But, to get HFCS, some enzymes, proteins which change things in your body, are added to change some of the glucose into fructose. The enzymes are alpha-amylase and Glucose amylase, from fungus (yes that's right) to break down those long chains of glucose. This eventually breaks the long chain starch into single glucoses which are then altered, again, using another enzyme, an isomerase, into some fructose. And, to all that, add a bunch of lab steps like, liquid chromatography, ion-exchange filtrations, and carbon adsorption, to remove impurities. The result is something which is "lab made", sweeter than table sugar, and the source of a bunch of studies showing an absolute link to obesity[10].

Don't get me wrong here. Beet and cane sugar also go through some steps in refining but end up as sucrose, not HFCS, and without much free fructose. Am I saying that fructose is toxic? No. But your body knows the difference between glucose, fructose, and sucrose. Don't believe those ads. Human metabolism is very, very specific. And evidence which we will go into does suggest that free fructose goes directly to your liver, makes it a fatty liver which is not as effective, and this contributes to something called "Metabolic Syndrome".

WHAT DOES HFCS DO TO ME?

So what's the proof that it makes a difference? What does it do to me? First we are going to give you the statistics on increased obesity, then the dietary studies with HFCS, and, finally, some heavy duty recent biochemical results including a discussion of something called "Metabolic Syndrome" (in the next chapter), sometimes also lumped in as pre-diabetes, but, it also includes pre-heart conditions as well. And a note to our readers; you can find and read the actual science publications by going to something called Pubmed. It's the online source for all science research articles. Just go to http://www.ncbi.nlm.nih.gov/pubmed

At the top there is a place to type in high fructose corn syrup and all the recent papers back to about 1970 or so will come up. Recently, most of us science types have also included online access to these papers and you can find that also at the top, usually right, to get the entire article in a PDF format. In some cases the abstract may be all you need to read. We know you are not all scientists so you can get the "bottom line" by reading the conclusion (last 2-3 sentences) of the abstract. I want you to try that now so you never again have to depend on sometimes false information on the internet or in TV ads. Try finding one of the papers listed in the "Reference" section of this book.

Papers go through a bunch of reviews by other scientists who would much rather publish their finding before you do. So, usually, the data in those publications is pretty accurate since it has been evaluated by a bunch of not so nice and very competitive folks. Some of the articles may state that HFCS has no bad effects. Be sure to check out the footnotes at the bottom of each article where they have to say who paid for their research. If it strikes you as a conflict of interest it could be.

ARE WE, IN FACT, GETTING FATTER?

We pulled these charts and stats from the CDC site (Communicable Disease Center) at http://www.cdc.gov/nchs/data/thestat/obesity_child07_08/obesity_child_07_08.htm (with permissions)

It is long, but, just check out the obesity site on the CDC homepage. In the Figure and Table, it is self-evident that obesity has increased from the 1970's to recent years and is not slowing. Obesity is defined by something called the Body Mass Index (BMI). You can calculate yours on any number of online sites. If you have not done this yet do it now. The BMI basically takes your weight and height and comes up with a number from around 18.5 – over 30. The break down is: underweight = 18.5 or less, normal weight = 18.5 – 24.9, overweight = 25 – 29.9, and obese =

over 30. This is for adults, and, if you are like me you have fought with and hovered around that number 25, especially if you are older.

The figure below plots the per cent increase in obesity (x—x) and HFCS consumption (●--●) over 30 years. You can see that they have increased together.

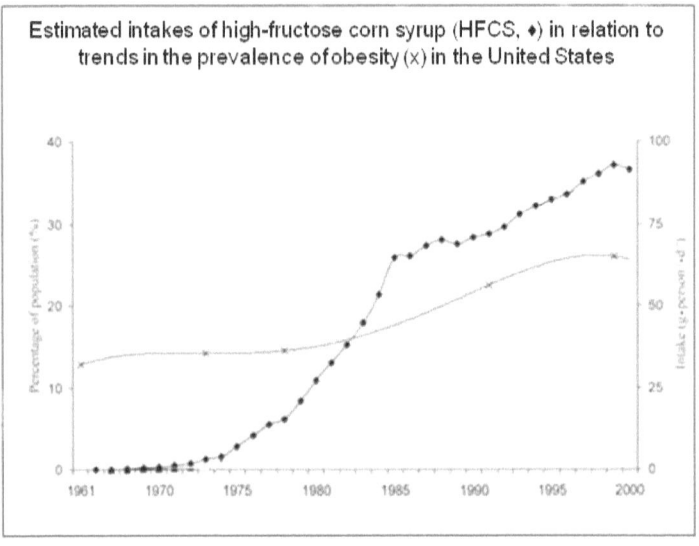

Adapted from **Fig. 9.2** Consumption of high fructose corn syrupPrimary source of sugar in the American diet, manufactured from corn starch and found in a variety of foods including soft drinks, popsicles and candy; linked to obesity. From Bray GA, Nielsen SJ, Popkin BM."Consumption of high-fructose corn syrup

in beverages may play a role in the epidemic of obesity" (2004) *American Journal of Clinical Nutrition*, 79:537.

Particularly disturbing is the increase in obesity in kids (they have a Table on the CDC site, too, shown below), even as young as 2-5 years of age (from 5% to 10%, or a doubling). Kids, aged 2-5, do not go out to restaurants by themselves nor do they go out alone and buy snacks. Parents and pre-schools do this to them. This means that one out of ten small kids are already obese and on their way to developing diabetes, heart problems and a host of other diseases associated with increased weight (ie., the "Metabolic Syndrome", discussed in the next chapter).

Prevalence of obesity among U.S. children and adolescents aged 2-19, for selected years 1963-1965 through 2007-2008

Age (in years)[1]	NHANES 1963-1965 1966-1970[2]	NHANES 1971-1974	NHANES 1976-1980	NHANES 1988-1994	NHANES 1999-2000	NHANES 2001-2002	NHANES 2003-2004	NHANES 2005-2006	NHANES 2007-2008
Total	([3])	5.0	5.5	10.0	13.9	15.4	17.1	15.5	16.9
2-5	([3])	5.0	5.0	7.2	10.3	10.6	13.9	11.0	10.4
6-11	4.2	4.0	6.5	11.3	15.1	16.3	18.8	15.1	19.6
12-19	4.6	6.1	5.0	10.5	14.8	16.7	17.4	17.8	18.1

1 Excludes pregnant women starting with 1971-1974. Pregnancy status not available for 1963-1965 and 1966-1970.
2 Data for 1963-1965 are for children aged 6-11; data for 1966-1970 are for adolescents aged 12-17, not 12-19 years.
3 Children aged 2-5 were not included in the surveys undertaken in the 1960s.
NOTE: Obesity defined as body mass index (BMI) greater than or equal to sex- and age-specific 95th percentile from the 2000 CDC Growth Charts.

From http://www.cdc.gov/nchs/data/hestat/obesity_child_07_08/obesity_child_07_08.htm

The picture gets even worse once they go to school. From ages 6-11 the increase from 1963 to 2008 was 4.2% to 19.6%. And, as teenagers, this does not stop (a 4.6 – 18.1% increase in obesity). Overall we are causing an epidemic of fat kids who will have a lifetime of health problems. Caloric intake has also increased by about 25% over the last 15 years. But, a 25% calorie increase could not, by itself cause this increase in obesity. This increase in obesity directly correlates with increased consumption of HFCS, artificial sweeteners, and use of plastics (see previous chapter). But, so what, so does the budget deficit. Both have increased greatly in recent times. How do we know if they are linked? And, what are the health effects on our kids and on us?

Just about everything has been blamed for this fat problem... overeating, too much fat, too much sugar, snacking, fast foods, and cholesterol. There have also been a host of really insane explanations. My favorite is the "hunter/gatherer" theory which states that we evolved to hunt and stuff ourselves in times of plenty when we were cave men. Well, guess what? The increase in weight really started in the 1970's and we were not cave men then.

Another is the "plenty" theory which is just another version of the "hunter/gatherer theory. This one says that we have a plentiful supply of food now which is tasty so we will eat more. The problem with this theory is that it assumes that we went from a third world country of starvation to a first world country from 1970 to present, and, you and I know that this is not true either. In fact, for those of you who are over 60, do you really remember vast starvation or lack of food in this country around 1970? I doubt it!

Finally, there is the theory of fast food, eating out at too many fast food places. Well, Coca Cola had been out for about 70 years by 1970, the first Jack in the Box opened in 1941, and McDonalds started in 1940. My favorite as a kid was Dairy Queen. It also began around 1940. I used to stop by there for ice cream every day after school as I walked home, back in 1960. In eighth grade I was already five foot two inches tall and weighed 90 lbs. I was not overweight even though I ate plenty of food and fast food every day!

Why do we harp on HFCS? Because, in the 1970's all of my favorite fast food restaurants and soft drinks began adding HFCS to their products, in place of sucrose. And, that is when we all started gaining weight.

In 1991 I had a sabbatical (fun Professor trip to a foreign country), to Holland to do some research, learn some new techniques, and take my two daughters to go to school in Europe for a semester. I had been wondering why kids and adults in the US where much heavier than their European counterparts. I thought that it was probably what everyone had said; the Europeans walked more, ate less, and did not have big desserts. Boy was I in for a surprise. At the lab that I worked in, at The University of Nijmegen, they told me they had all had only coffee and a roll for breakfast before they got in. OK, same as me. But we had a morning break for coffee and sweet rolls at 10 am and then, at <u>precisely</u> noon (they are Dutch, after all), we had a very large meal consisting of meat, potatoes, a vegetable, maybe soup, bread, milk, and a dessert. About three hours after that, at around 3-4 pm, we broke again for afternoon tea which also included something sweet, like one of those beautiful cakes you see in the magazines.

So I asked them what they ate for dinner. The Dutch eat early compared to southern Europeans who are famous for those midnight dinners. At around 7 pm or so, they ate a dinner of meats, cheeses, breads and vegetables. I was a dinner guest at several houses and the meals were not small. But there was a difference. They did not snack between meals, did not eat fast foods, and all foods were prepared and not what we would call "convenience foods". But, they did eat jarred vegetables and fruits (the Dutch are into recycling and do not usually "can" things). At that time they also did not go to fast food places although they loved to go out to restaurants and eat huge quantities of Dutch or Indonesian foods and beer. So anyway my idea of their eating less or not eating fats or desserts went down the drain. In fact, I found out that the incidence of gall bladder removal was high in Holland due to the excess consumption of high fat foods, like cheese.

When I returned, I told my husband that it was something in the actual foods that we eat and not, strictly, caloric consumption. Although I do have to add that people who eat fast food, or who drink one of those supersized soft drinks are just plain consuming more calories than they are burning. One other thing, the idea that the Dutch get more exercise by walking and riding bikes is greatly exaggerated. I think we should increase our exercise here, don't get me wrong. But, the Dutch are not all marathon runners and I would not attribute their thinness to more exercise. It's the food, plain and simple. But this is all anecdotal isn't it? Where's the scientific proof? Why do I really blame HFCS? Or, as people in my class will ask me, "Is it the extra calories or the HFCS". The answer is yes.

FAT RATS AND PEOPLE TOO

OK, what do you mean by "yes"? I asked two questions. Later in this chapter I will explain that the answer is "yes" to both questions. The HFCS is, itself, causing obesity, and, we eat more calories because fructose does not signal "full" to the brain. You doubt the last answer? This is the test I give to my class and what I want you to try now. Drink a 24 oz soft drink that contains HFCS and see if you can finish it in 30 minutes. Now, the next day, go get two 12 oz bottles of Coca Cola in the glass bottles, from Mexico, and pour those into the 24 oz glass. Be sure that the bottles say "cane sugar" (ie., sucrose) on the label. Now try to drink that in 30 minutes. When my students try this they have a very hard time finishing the soft drinks made with cane sugar (sucrose and not HFCS). They say that they feel too full and have to force themselves to finish the drink. As I will discuss below, glucose sends messages of "fullness" to the brain while fructose does not.

WHAT CONTROLS MY APPETITE?

When you were a baby your mom or dad held up that spoon of yellow glop from the baby food jar and said, "Ummmm! Maybe it's the smile or maybe you are just tired of the milk all the time, by then. Or, maybe, you notice that the rest of the family isn't just taking their meals from a bottle. At any rate you taste it and, if it is not off your scale of acceptance, you take some in, mostly all over your face, but, eventually into your body. These learned signals, very early in life, teach you to accept certain foods and reject others. Sometimes, once we leave home, we learn, as adults, to like other types of foods. However, there is a certain range of acceptance by all humans which protects them from ingestion of poisons. Taste is a combination of both taste and smell. And, it is mostly smell.

We have taste buds with receptors, on our tongues, which can sense 5 types of tastes; salty, sour, umami, bitter, and sweet.

Receptor is just another name for a protein which sits on the surface of a cell and "detects" the taste. Each of these is spread out all over the tongue, contrary to what some think. They are not grouped by taste type.

Salty allows us to determine if we are getting enough ions like sodium. Sour can perk up the appetite but also help determine if the food is spoiled. Umami is also called the glutamate taste system. Glutamate, mimicked by monosodium glutamate or MSG, is an amino acid so this receptor is for that yummy chicken soup flavor. In other words, to be sure we get enough protein. Bitter taste is the most important one and we have two signal systems for bitter. One determines if something is so bitter that it might be a poison, while another signal system tells us that a certain amount is OK, like the caffeine in coffee, as an example.

Sweet taste receptors come in at least two forms, one big receptor for the natural sugar, sucrose, which you have seen in the figure shown above. Another type of receptor can detect trehalose and some of the other artificial sweeteners. So right away you know that the taste receptors for sweeteners can be different. I will discuss artificial sweeteners below at the end of the chapter. The fructose receptor is different than the glucose receptor. The glucose receptors are on brain cells to signal fullness and on pancreas cells to signal insulin release, among many other places in your body.

You can find a great popular set of articles on all the sensory systems in a journal called Nature[11], by checking that Pubmed site that I told you about. It's easy to read and has great pictures.

Smell is really what we use to detect food. That's why real estate agents tell you to bake cookies before your open house. You can go into a cafeteria and, once you smell the turkey and stuffing, you will have a bunch of Thanksgiving memories, some cooking, some washing dishes, and, some football. Food smells are intricately stored in your memories of events. We can smell about 100,000 different odors, have at least 1000 different smell receptors in our nasal cavity (nose), and they combine signals so that we can smell over a range of 0.1 micromolar (abbreviated µM) to 10 millimolar (mM), a 100,000 fold range. We can also smell many things at a time. Smell, taste, and what we are taught come together so that we like or hate certain foods. There's a lot of culture mixed in too. Japanese generally do not like cheese, the Dutch love it. Americans love peanut butter and jelly sandwiches which are disgusting to the Dutch, who put their peanuts on meat (peanut satay). We love chocolate for dessert while the Dutch eat a version as a sandwich for lunch. But, we all love sweets.

This love of the sweet taste probably came from very early mankind, while searching for foods that would provide them with energy. While the protein from their hunts would keep them going for a longer time, the sweet honey, stolen from hives, gave them a quick boost. But, until recent times the consumption of sugar and honey was small and supplies were hard to come by. And, obesity was something that only the very wealthy experienced.

OK, But, What Controls my Appetite?

Sorry, I got carried away up there. Right, now back to your question. The answer is Leptin, peptide YY, neuropeptide Y, and Ghrelin. Say what? OK, those are some of the hormones that we know about so far that affect appetite. You lost me.

We scientist types are just beginning to determine what controls your appetite on a biochemical level. Leptin was the first hormone to be discovered. It is a small protein which is produced by fat cells (also called adipose cells) and regulates the amount of fat that you have and your general energy needs[12-16] Leptin is called a neuroendocrine hormone because it sends information to the brain appetite centers to control food intake and fat storage. The blood level of leptin is directly proportional to the amount of fat in your body[21]. There are a few people around the world who have no leptin and were obese. When given leptin their weight dropped[17]. But, most people do not have a lack of leptin so that, most likely, is not the cause of their obesity.

Leptin binds to leptin receptors (those proteins which recognize it and are found on leptin target types of cells). These are mostly in a region of the brain which controls appetite and metabolism, the hypothalamus. Leptin inhibits your appetite by counteracting another hormone called neuropeptide Y, a potent brain protein which stimulates feeding by signaling to the brain and gut. The absence of leptin leads to uncontrolled food intake, and, causes obesity[21]. In other words, leptin signals to the brain that you are full while neuropeptide Y signals that it is time to eat[22].

Ghrelin and peptide YY are two gastro-intestinal (stomach/digestive system) protein hormones which circulate around the body. Ghrelin stimulates appetite and food consumption and peptide YY suppresses your appetite and food intake[23,24]. Ghrelin was the first circulating (in the blood) hormone discovered which stimulates hunger. Peptide YY, on the other hand, is released from the ileum and colon in response to eating. It reduces your appetite[24]. In other words, these two hormones have opposing roles in your body.

HFCS messes up the levels of all of these hormones in your body. So HFCS helps you consume more calories but also re-directs your metabolism to store more fat. In fact, the free fructose that is in HFCS goes mostly to the liver where it is changed, by Central Metabolism, to fat. So, yes, it's the extra calories and the HFCS. HFCS sabotages your appetite control center so you want to eat more, and, the HFCS is changed to fat easier. Don't take my word for it, go to the actual Pubmed papers listed in the Reference section and read them. Unless you become more proactive about your own health you will continue to have to trust those TV ads.

So let me summarize:

1. Leptin = from fat cells (called adipocytes), goes to brain and suppresses appetite and controls amount of fat.

2. Neuropeptide Y= from the brain, it stimulates appetite

3. Ghrelin = from the digestive system, it circulates through the blood and stimulates your appetite

4. Peptide YY = also from the digestive system, it suppresses your appetite

So those are <u>some</u> of the hormones that control what you eat, how much, and how much fat your body has. I have included them here because the studies below clearly show that HFCS messes with their ability to control your appetite.

A Couple of Research Results

In your Pubmed search online (you are now experts, so find this article online now and read along with me) you will find an article from 2004, first author, Karen L. Teff[18]. The title of this article is, "Dietary Fructose Reduces Circulating Insulin and Leptin, Attenuates Postprandial Suppression of Ghrelin, and Increases Triglycerides in Women". Let me translate that; "<u>Eating fructose reduces blood levels of insulin</u> (insulin stimulates glucose uptake into cells, so now your blood sugar is high and you could be pre-diabetic) <u>and leptin</u> (the hormone that controls fat, so now you get fatter easier<u>), reduces the drop in ghrelin after a meal</u> (remember, ghrelin stimulates your appetite, so you are now still hungry), <u>and increases fat</u> (we scientists call fats triglycerides) <u>in women</u>".

Does that say it all or what? I like to start my class on nutrition with this article because it shows results with real <u>human</u> ladies. And, at the end of this chapter, I discuss the fat rats. That study only shows increases in tummy fat with lady rats so those who support HFCS jump on those results, saying there was no difference found in weight. This is true, but, only for the boy rats. Us ladies just cannot eat the HFCS and keep a trim waistline.

This first study[18] tested 12 normal women, aged 19-33 with a body mass index of 19.8 – 26.7. In other words, they were not obese. They consumed 3 meals per day with about 1200-2000 calories per day. If you want to know exactly what they ate check out the second page of the article under Diet. Meals were 55% carbohydrates, 30% fat, and 15% protein in all cases. The only difference was that one group had 30% of their calories from HFCS and the other group had their 30% from glucose-sweetened beverages. What happened? Well, HFCS consumption reduced insulin by 65%, reduced leptin by 33%, increased ghrelin by around 40%, and triglycerides (fats) by around 20%. Translated that means that you can drink a 24 oz soft drink with HFCS in it and still feel hungry, even though you have taken in about 300 calories. And, you will have more fat floating around in your blood.

The next study, also listed on Pubmed, is from 2008, with Michael M. Swarbrick[19] as the first author. The title is, "Consumption of fructose-sweetened beverages for 10 weeks increases postprandial triacylglycerol and apolipoprotein-B concentrations in overweight and obese women". Postprandial means after your meal.

This article sounds pretty much the same as the other one, but was longer (10 weeks), and also measured something called apolipoprotein-B (ApoB). This little protein is found mixed up with some fat as a big complex in your blood. Fat does not get carried around very well in the blood so it needs a carrier. So does cholesterol, another type of fat. Fats are carried through your blood to your cells by these big complexes. You have heard the terms "good and bad cholesterol". This actually refers to the big complexes with fats, proteins and cholesterol all in a ball. They provide the transport systems for fats to get out of the blood and into the cells.

We scientists classify them by whether they float better or not, their density. You may have read this on your blood tests as HDL (high density lipoprotein, lipo for lipid or fat, high meaning high density), LDL (low density lipoprotein), and VLDL (very low density lipoprotein). HDL is what you call "good cholesterol" because that complex takes the cholesterol to the liver to be broken down instead of coating your arteries. VLDL contains the ApoB, one of the protein "carriers", and so, when you consume more fructose, you get more bad cholesterol, or cholesterol which floats around in the blood and causes your arteries to clog up. This is known as the "Metabolic Syndrome" which is discussed in the next chapter. So, not only can HFCS make you fat, it can also make you very sick.

I want to warn you, there are a number of people who fault the studies above. After all, why compare HFCS with glucose when the alternative is sucrose (table sugar, half glucose and half fructose), not glucose. Several studies have shown that HFCS is not different than sucrose. Let's see the latest study.

FAT RATS

I want to end this chapter section on HFCS with the last study, published in 2010, with Miriam E. Bocarsly[20] as first author (again check out Pubmed, online, and read along with me). First of all, this study has been the source of contention among those supporting HFCS. They only looked at the left chart for boy rats. Let's look at the lady rats on the right. If they eat Ad libitum (meaning whenever they want), it is pretty apparent that the ladies drinking the HFCS have fatter tummies (abdominal fat) than those drinking sucrose. Yes, this is the HFCS vs sucrose study that was needed.

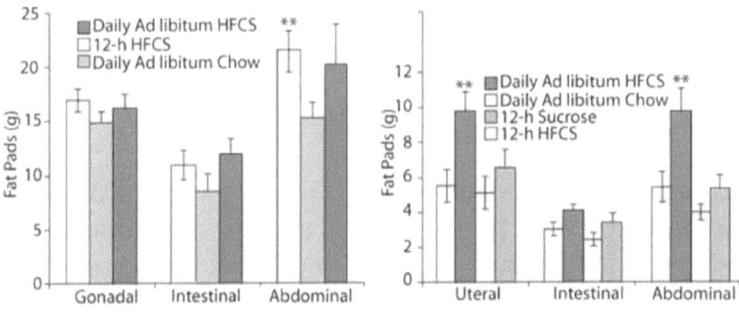

Fig. 9.3 Fat accumulation by rats. Left panel: Males fed either 24- or 12-h HFCS diets. Right panel: Females maintained on 24-h access to HFCS and chow.

http://www.cfsan.fda.gov/~dms/fdsugar.html
Bray, G.A., S.J. Nielsen, and B.M. Popkin. (2004). Consumption of high-fructose corn syrup in beverages may play a role in the epidemic
Warner, M. (2006). Does this goo make you groan? New York Times, July 2, Section 3, pp. 1, 8, 9.
Bocarsly, M.E., et al. (2010). High-fructose corn syrup causes characteristics of obesity in rats: Increased body weight, body fat and triglyceride levels. Pharmacol. Biochem. Behav. Feb 26. [Epub ahead of print]

In fact, this even doubled in size (measured as grams of fat pads) from 5 to 10 grams. This does not sound like a lot but it is to a rat! We ladies, human or rat, just can't take in HFCS without messing with our waistlines. And that's a serious problem because tummy size directly correlates with increased incidence of "Metabolic Syndrome". Obviously, unlike those TV ads, your body does know the difference between table sugar (sucrose) and HFCS. And this has serious consequences to your health. In the studies listed above, the normal rats and women (normal or obese) who ate or drank HFCS, had higher blood fat levels (triglycerides), gained weight, had less insulin effects, changed the ability of their blood to transport and get rid of cholesterol, and were still hungry.

How does this happen and why? HFCS does not signal to cells that they have enough energy. Fructose is not the same as glucose. Cells have glucose receptors which are very specific, and, that is the natural "fullness" system of your body. Fructose does not substitute for this. Therefore, you tend to eat more, and, then, your liver has to figure out what to do with all that fructose. What does that do? In the next chapter we describe something called "Metabolic Syndrome", and, describe exactly what HFCS is doing to contribute to this serious health risk.

But I Drink Diet Sodas!

Artificial sweeteners were first introduced with the synthesis of saccharin in 1879[25]. Initially it was used as a sucrose substitute for those with diabetes. During World War II there was a sugar shortage and people also wanted to be thinner so, thus, began the addition of artificial sweeteners to foods and soft drinks. Diet coke started in 1983 and now almost all foods have some form of "diet" version with artificial sweeteners added.

The ones now used are shown below, along with the commercial names. Saccharine is about 300 times sweeter than sucrose and was the only one used, mostly by diabetics who wanted to limit glucose, up until about 1965. It's hard to say if people just wanted to be thinner or if there was an aggressive ad crusade but other sweeteners followed and now you can find at least three on any restaurant table. Soft drinks often use a combination of several depending on the taste panel tests for the product. Currently there are about 4000 products on the market that contain an artificial sweetener, including, the flavored varieties of Pedialyte (for infants). We, of course, consume diet sodas all the time, so, does this help us to keep our weight down?

You would think so since most, except aspartame, have no calories and those diet sodas are calorie free. The studies in the 1970's with 31,940 women showed that saccharin use was actually associated with weight gain[25]. Another study of a cross-section of children and youth found that diet soda drinkers had elevated BMI. This is not due to any special effects of the artificial sweeteners on metabolism. Unlike fructose they are not damaging (except aspartame). However, individuals who drink diet sodas, it was found, had a higher caloric intake because sweet tastes, whether real or artificial enhance appetite.

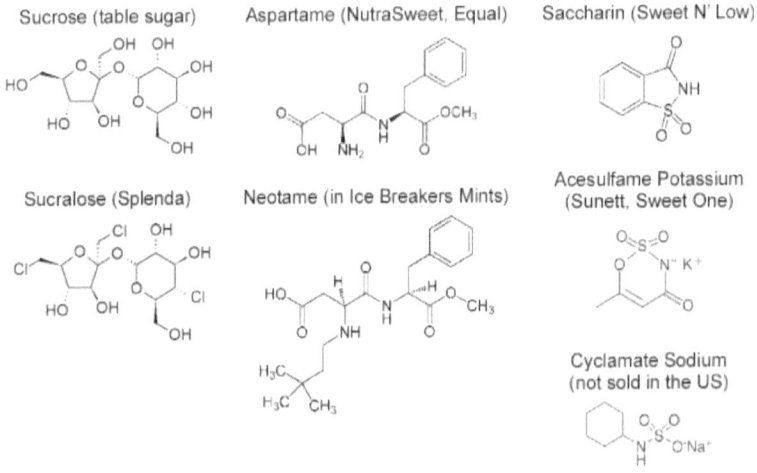

Sucrose (table sugar)

Aspartame (NutraSweet, Equal)

Saccharin (Sweet N' Low)

Sucralose (Splenda)

Neotame (in Ice Breakers Mints)

Acesulfame Potassium
(Sunett, Sweet One)

Cyclamate Sodium
(not sold in the US)

Aspartame, Acesulfame Potassium, and saccharine are all associated with increased appetite.

A chart of weight gain along with the introduction of artificial sweeteners definitely shows that when new products were introduced the weight gain just kept on climbing [25-27]. It does not do any good to drink a ton of soft drinks with artificial sweeteners because, once again, they do not signal "full" to the brain, do not satisfy your energy needs and leave you still hungry. So you eat more and gain more weight.

ASPARTAME, A TOXIC SWEETENER

Wow! You called it toxic! You are right, there are not many things in this book that I will refer to as toxic. But, aspartame is one of them. Aspartame was discovered (synthesized from chemicals) in 1965 by a scientist who was trying to make a new ulcer drug. Let's look at the structure shown above for aspartame (also called NutraSweet or Equal). Everything from the NH to the right is the amino acid, phenylalanine. Everything left of the NH (in the middle) is the amino acid, aspartic acid. Unlike all the other artificial sweeteners, aspartame is metabolized in your cells and, also, can cross the barrier between the blood and your brain, called the blood/brain barrier (BBB). In 2002 aspartame was further altered to create neotame, which is 7000 times sweeter than sucrose, and, has a methanol added.

The problem lies in the fact that aspartame can get broken down to its components, aspartic acid, methanol, and phenylalanine. In fact, people with the genetic disease, phenylketonuria (PKU), should not use aspartame as it will cause further brain damage. A warning sign should appear on all foods with aspartame. It is found in most diet sodas.

In one case aspartame was also found to cause fibromyalgia, a chronic pain condition which was cured once the aspartame was removed from the patient's diet[27].

The phenylalanine which comes from the aspartame gets changed in the brain to tyrosine, another amino acid which is a component of neurotransmitters such as dopamine, epinephrine, and norepinephrine. These are vital neurotransmitters in the brain involved in brain development, memory and what we call neuro-cognitive functions (learning). In sensitive individuals the ingestion of aspartame has caused migraine headaches, insomnia and even seizures. Defects in dopamine have been linked to tics, obsessive compulsive disorder, Parkinson's Disease, and ADHD[26]. Aspartame is found in Diet Coke and Diet Pepsi, children's vitamins, flavored Pedialytes, and about 6000 others foods. Until further work is done, this product should never be given to infants or children or pregnant women.

We hope that you have learned some things about the food you eat and what toxic substances are present which can make you sick. All of this can lead to something called, Metabolic Syndrome.

METABOLIC SYNDROME

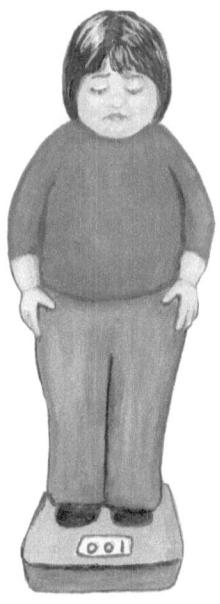

<u>What Happens if I Keep Eating It?</u>

What happens if you continue to consume large quantities of HFCS? Or, those leached plastics that raise your estrogen levels? You have examined the research for yourself, now, by using the Pubmed online search. You know, for example, that if you consume large quantities of HFCS, like what is in many soft drinks, you will gain weight. But, is that necessarily so bad? Maybe your family is large anyway, or you are not really that overweight, or have a borderline BMI of around 25, like me. So what, you are young and healthy, right? Maybe, or maybe not. Clearly, research shows that the consumption of HFCS and being overweight can lead to something referred to as "Metabolic Syndrome". This is actually a collection of unhealthy states which have only recently been lumped together.

In this chapter we want to describe what Metabolic Syndrome is and tell you about the growing concern that we have for you and your kids.

First, what is Metabolic Syndrome? It has been called a bunch of things over the year including, Reaven's syndrome, Insulin resistant syndrome, and diabesity. But, none of these really fit because, the insulin/diabetes effects were not all that was seen in people, and who cares about someone named Reaven. He was the guy who, around 1988, named the condition as "symptoms syndrome X", but doctors now usually refer to it as Metabolic Syndrome. And this condition is increasing, even in children. The CDC report shows that around 34% of the adult population now has Metabolic Syndrome[1-3]. An estimated 1 million 12-19-year-old kids in the United States now have Metabolic Syndrome, and, this number is growing! We may outlive our kids!

There are five signs of Metabolic Syndrome, and, you have it if you have three of the signs. These are (not listed in any order of importance):

1. Abdominal (tummy or waist line) Obesity

   No one wants to be fat, but, the type of fat around the waist is the most dangerous. And you saw that a diet high in HFCS caused weight gain around the tummy (abdominal fat, sometimes abbreviated as VAT for visceral adipose tissue). In fact, the studies with HFCS or fructose *vs.* glucose diets often do not show increased total weight gain over the short periods of the studies, just a gain in the waistline (VAT) compared to subcutaneous (overall) fat (SAT)[4-6]. This type of fat is a predictor of heart disease, type 2 diabetes, and, elevated blood pressure.

There is no doubt that the average waistline has increased. This is probably why those hip hugger jeans are so popular. You can avoid thinking about your waist line when your pants hug your hips. In fact, we have shown you, in the first chapter that the size charts for some of the popular sewing pattern companies have become bigger to compensate for our increased weight around the waist! You may have noticed this trend in clothing sizes at your favorite store.

The average waist size as of 2008 for the American man was 40 inches, a 5 inch increase over 40 years[2]. For American women this is even worse, the average waist size being 37 inches, with an increase of 7 inches over the last 40 years. Some suggest that it is better to look at the waist to hip ratio, optimal being less than 0.8 for women and 0.9 for men. We scientists don't know why a diet high in HFCS causes more weight gain around the waist. But, the American Heart Association says it is more dangerous than normal weight gain. They call it the "apple" or "pear" shape figure.

In this 5 point test, mark <u>one point</u> if your waist is greater than 35 inches for women and 40 inches for men. But, most doctors would make those 37 inches for men and 32 inches for women. And, I only have one inch to spare, by those counts.

2. Elevated Blood Triglycerides

In the previous chapter we showed you that a diet high in fructose or HFCS caused elevated blood triglycerides. In fact, this was seen in almost all of the studies in both rats and humans, and, was one of the first things to be observed, sometimes even without a total weight gain.

So what is a triglyceride? When you eat a meal which is high in fats those fats get changed (digested) in the stomach and intestines. Let's take a look at that. In the figure below I show you a picture of a type of triglyceride (tri for three long strings, and "glyceride" for the glycerol that they are attached to).

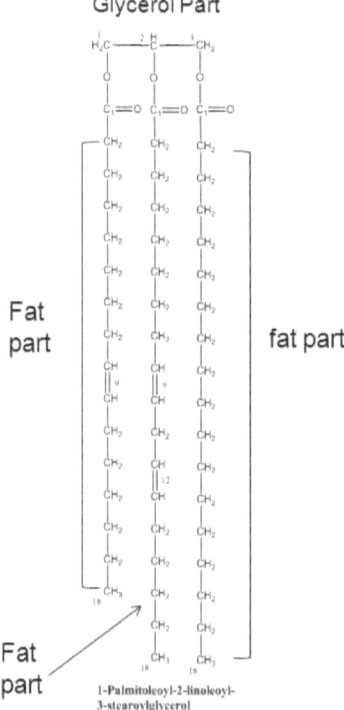

Glycerol Part

Fat part

Fat part

fat part

1-Palmitoleoyl-2-linoleoyl-3-stearoylglycerol

They do not all look like this since the "fat part" changes with your diet. For example, if you eat a bunch of saturated fats the long strings hanging down on the structure shown above have CH_2-CH_2 with only one line to connect them. This is called a single bond and it means that the two carbon atoms (C's) are connected by a single bond. Double bonds (CH=CH) are called unsaturated. If you have more than one of these in the long string, like the middle one in the figure (noted with a 9 and 12) then we call this polyunsaturated. If it is an omega fat, like in fish oils, that means there is a CH=CH so many C's in from the end. Take a look at the figure and check out the far left "fat part" with the 9 next to it. If you wanted to say what kind of omega fat it was you would now count in from the end, numbered as 16 in the figure, but, counting backwards, the first CH=CH that you come to would be number 7. So this "fat part" is a 7-omega fat. We all know that unsaturated fats and omega fats are better than saturated fats. This is because they are broken down easier and do not accumulate as much in your arteries.

When a CH=CH is made it can either make a straight string or a bent one. The trans fats have double bonds which make a straight string and this causes them to look like saturated fats to the cell. You have learned to avoid trans fats because, when they go into your cells they trap cholesterol, like saturated fats do, and this raises cellular cholesterol levels. Now, food labels have to report the levels of trans fats and most producers have adjusted their procedures to come up with a product that does not contain any trans fats.

In the figure above I have shown you the glycerol with three connected fatty acids. These long strings of CH_2-CH_2-CH_2- etc. do not dissolve in water. They are the "fat part" of this "thing". So when you eat them in your diet they have to travel through the blood by attaching themselves to "Carriers". You learned what the names of these carriers were, LDL, VLDL, and HDL.

You learned in a previous chapter that these became elevated when on a HFCS diet. Fructose is not used in the same way that glucose is, it is changed to fat. Fructose has six carbons which get cut into two 3-carbon "things" which make that glycerol for the triglycerides. Glucose gets into central metabolism in another way and does not do this. If you can't get rid of the fat, this will show on your blood test as elevated blood triglycerides (sometimes abbreviated as TGA). If you have fasting levels of triglycerides in your blood test of above 150 milligrams (mg) per deciliter (dL, or 100 milliliters), then this is too high and you should give yourself <u>one point</u> on the Metabolic Syndrome test.

3. <u>Low HDL (high density lipoprotein)</u>

What? How about my just plain cholesterol levels? Where do they come in? If you have a copy, take a look at your latest blood work from your last yearly physical. It is very confusing isn't it? Sometimes it says LDL (<u>l</u>ow <u>d</u>ensity <u>l</u>ipoprotein) and sometimes LDL or HDL cholesterol. That just means the amount of cholesterol in the HDL *vs* the LDL "carrier complex". The really important figure is the total cholesterol in the blood divided by the amount of cholesterol in the HDL component. So if your profile does not give this number then find your total cholesterol level, say 240, and divide that by the HDL number, say 57. If your number is less than 5.0 then you are OK. So, really, your HDL cholesterol needs to be higher than 50.

What does all this mean? Well, cholesterol is in your diet all the time so even if you fasted the night before some will be around and will depend on if you ate a steak the night before. They don't want just that information. The physicians want to know if your body can deal with it or if it is going to stay around and clog up your arteries. The carrier HDL grabs the cholesterol and takes it to the liver to be broken down to less harmful stuff. So, the more HDL, the better you are.

The LDL can't do this for you. It just drags that cholesterol all over the place and stuffs it into those cracks in your arteries. You read about the effects of HFCS on HDL and LDL levels, in a previous chapter. It was not good. The levels of both LDL and VLDL (very low density lipoprotein) went up, and so would your "junk" cholesterol.

The consumption of HFCS has been shown to increase liver fat accumulation (something called steatosis) from 5% in a control person to 25% in someone eating HFCS[4]. So, over time, your liver cannot deal with getting rid of the cholesterol or triglycerides because it is not functioning correctly. This leads to cardiovascular problems.

Your HDL level should be greater than 50. If you are a man and your HDL is lower than 40 mg/dL, or, a women with HDL lower than 50 mg/dL, give yourself <u>one point.</u>

4. <u>High Blood Pressure</u>

    High blood pressure is one of those weird things. It can be linked to HFCS, or not, linked to obesity, or not, or linked to genetics, or not. There are people who regularly do triathlons who have high blood pressure, and, people who are very obese who do not have high blood pressure, or not.

    Blood is pumped through your arteries and capillaries by your heart. And you have to have that blood pumped correctly to get oxygen and nutrients to cells and organs. We all know this. Blood pressure refers to the force that the blood has on your blood vessel walls as it goes through your body. If your blood vessels are getting clogged up, from fat accumulation on the blood vessel walls, the pumping would be harder to do, like a clogged drain pipe. The reading for blood pressure has two numbers which are given as the larger over the smaller, like 120/70. The first number (the higher one, a systolic reading) is called the systolic pressure, the force exerted as your heart contracts (the lub of the lub dub), the second number (lower, a diastolic reading) is the one taken as your heart relaxes. Any kind of pressure is usually given as millimeters of mercury, mm Hg (Hg is the atomic chart abbreviation for mercury).

    When you visit the doctor's office a nurse will strap a cuff on your arm and use a pump to exert pressure on your arm then this will be attached to a pressure reader, in mm Hg. High blood pressure would be a systolic pressure of above 140 mm and/or a diastolic pressure of higher than 90 mm Hg. High blood pressure is called the silent killer because there aren't very many symptoms. But, you are slowly overworking your heart and it could be a sign that you have a clogged blood vessel somewhere. It is much worse than a high cholesterol level and should be taken very seriously.

And, to be fair, a lot more than HFCS contributes to elevated blood pressure, like a high salt diet or just plain bad genetics. But, it is almost always linked to weight gain if there is no genetic component. Most people who have high blood pressure can lower it by losing weight. And that is where the HFCS comes in, in a bad way. But, as they say, "that's not all". Some very recent work shows that the fructose receptor on cells interacts with the salt transporters on those same cells. And this alters blood pressure.[7] If you have blood pressure which is greater than 140/90 mm Hg, or, if you take blood pressure medicine, give yourself one point.

5.   High Blood Glucose (also called blood sugar)

If your physician asks you to take a blood glucose test this could be done in several ways. Remember that blood sugar means blood glucose because 99.99% of the blood sugar is glucose and those measurements are for glucose and nothing else. Our bodies have evolved to use only glucose in central metabolism and the brain has glucose receptors, not fructose receptors. The pancreas releases insulin in response to blood glucose, not fructose. If you cannot control this you may have diabetes. We all know that pre-diabetic individuals show a lack of sensitivity to insulin. This is the hormone released from the pancreas to signal cells to take up glucose so that the blood level of glucose can be controlled. Individuals who are pre-diabetic will not be able to clear their blood glucose levels after drinking a liquid glucose drink.

Maybe you have a family history of diabetes. In that case you may take two types of tests at the doctor's office, a general blood glucose test after fasting overnight, and, a glucose clearance test, after drinking a glucose solution, which would tell you how fast the glucose got out of your blood after one big dose. No matter what, it is absolutely critical that your blood glucose remain someplace between 70 – 100 mg/dL over the general time period. Too high blood glucose is called hyperglycemia and too low is called hypoglycemia. People with diabetes can die from either.

I know that we usually think of diabetes as high blood glucose/sugar. But, in order to control the blood glucose levels an individual may have to take insulin as a shot. Insulin is a hormone from the pancreas. It tells cells to take glucose out of the blood and into the individual cell that can recognize the insulin as a signal. This has the nice effect of lowering blood glucose, but, if the blood glucose goes too low something called "insulin shock" occurs. The diabetic individual may become too hypoglycemic and this can cause death. One of the big areas of research by labs and drug companies is to try to create a better way to detect changes in blood glucose so that the insulin would be given to the diabetic person in a more controlled manner. You may know someone who has an insulin pump for this purpose.

How does insulin work? Actually the pancreas can make two different protein hormones and release them into the blood when glucose levels are high (insulin) or low (glucagon). The pancreas is one of those organs that you just can't live without. It has both digestive and glucose-controlling functions. The chief reason that you need to control glucose is that the brain generally only uses glucose for energy. There are sensors in the brain and in the pancreas which are there to be sure that your brain gets enough glucose. Remember that when we say blood sugar we mean glucose because that is 99.99% of the sugar in the blood.

You may not be diabetic but most of us have experienced a big drop in blood glucose maybe after exercising or when going without food for a long time. You may have felt shaky, tired, or even light headed. This was all due to your brain telling your body that the blood glucose was too low and that it (the brain) needed some more glucose for its food/energy source.

Your body takes care of this in several ways. First, the liver stores glucose as long chains called glycogen. When the liver "reads" the low glucose signal some enzymes break down those long glucose chains to individual glucose and that is released from the liver cells into the blood to return glucose levels back to normal. This is our first line of defense against low blood sugar. Athletes who want to run a long distance need that blood sugar so they do what is called "carb loading". This means that they eat a lot of carbohydrates so that the liver can be stuffed with glycogen. This serves as their quick blood sugar source while running. So everyone really needs a healthy liver.

When blood glucose levels drop your pancreas releases glucagon. The glucagon goes through the blood to whichever cells have the ability to recognize it (have glucagon receptors). Once the glucagon gets to its target cell, a bunch of signals tell that cell to break down the stored glucose (starch or glycogen) and release it into the blood so that the blood glucose level can get back up to normal levels. The opposite happens after you eat or when glucose levels go up in the blood. Then the pancreas releases insulin to bind to its cell targets and this signals that cell to take glucose into the cell from the blood. The glucose is then stored back into starch or glycogen. This is not always a totally smooth cycle so you may get shaky for awhile until things get back to normal.

Consuming too much fructose has been shown to cause us to become less sensitive to insulin[8].

This signal system, between glucagon and insulin, is what keeps your blood glucose level under control. If you are diabetic, this control is gone. If your blood glucose level is above 100 mg/ dL give yourself <u>one point.</u>

All of these things lead to stress on your body. Recently we scientists have noticed that stress in the pancreas leads to chronic inflammation. In order to determine the inflammatory state of an individual the lab will test your blood for something called C-reactive protein. When you have inflammation some of your cells die and they spill out a fat called phosphocholine[3,8,9]. In addition bacteria also release C-protein and this is a sign of an infection. C-reactive protein (the C is for choline) binds to choline and so it is increased when you have inflammation in some part of your body. This eventually gets into the blood and it will be detected by a blood test as higher than normal. It is used in labs to determine if an individual has an increased risk of diabetes, hypertension, or cardiovascular disease. Normal levels are around 10 mg/L or less and an individual has high C-reactive protein above 40 mg/L. If you have high C-protein this is another indicator of Metabolic Syndrome since heart disease and diabetes both have an inflammatory component.

Some individuals with Metabolic Syndrome also have a high risk of blood clotting due to high clotting factors in the blood. These can also be measured by a lab blood test to measure levels of blood clotting factors.

If you have 3 points or more, using the above criteria, you probably have Metabolic Syndrome. What does this mean? It means that you have a much greater risk of getting type 2 diabetes and/or heart disease. And, this is happening at a younger and younger age.

You can avoid all of this by following the guidelines in this book.

1. Avoid things with high fructose corn syrup or corn syrup in them using the list we have given you.

2. Avoid artificial sweeteners and keep sugar and salt consumption low by SLOWLY decreasing their consumption.

3. Watch the containers that your food comes in and never ever use plastic baby bottles.

4. Read the labels!

This all sounds so simple but really needs a plan.
If you have a plan "YOU CAN DO IT".

YOU CAN DO IT!
HERE'S HOW

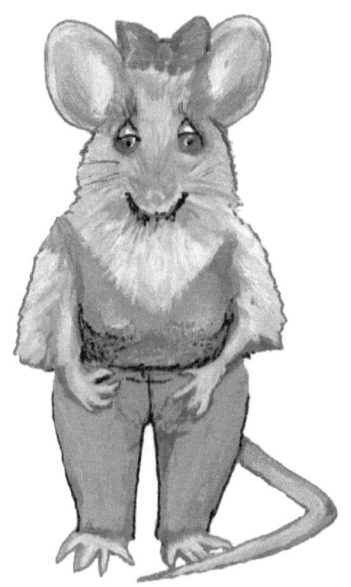

We realize that this is a lot to take in for some people. Some of us have been just going into the store and buying whatever looks appetizing without much thought of the content. We have been depending on the Food and Drug Administration to have our best interests in mind. But just like in every other organization, including our families, the FDA (and we) has compromised the ideal for a less demanding substitute. We try to take the easier way for everything. If the meal is already half prepared, then it is less stressful for the busy working mother. We mothers have gotten tired of everyone depending on us to put a good meal on the table for the whole family after we have spent a long day at work solving problems and fighting traffic. We even ask the kids what they want for dinner. Of course, they are going to say pizza or hotdogs or something they saw advertised on TV. Or, you know, that if you just drive through a fast food place you don't even have to prepare anything. And it is cheap and includes a toy.

When we were kids, our mom put a balanced meal on everyone's plate and we were expected to eat everything because there were starving children in some far away country. There still are.

The point is this. You are in charge of making choices for good reasons. You are the adult with more education and better judgment. You can teach your children what is healthy to eat and what will make them live longer and be stronger. You can tell them why. And now, with the internet, you can look a lot of this information up. You only have to decide to take the time.

I know, you wonder, what time? Well, we have made it easy for you. Once you follow these steps and use the food lists in the Appendix it will become easier. You will remember which brands to buy. And they are increasing every year! And the best thing is some of the cheapest brands, like "Great Value" already took out the high fructose corn syrup. So here is our plan:

Start small. Carry the list of substitutes with you to the grocery store, if you have to. Otherwise just put the brand name on your list so you can have that information when you do that usual evening rush through the store. If someone at home asks what happened to their favorite brand of something you can tell them why you changed it to a brand without high fructose corn syrup. If you do it slowly, maybe some will not even notice the difference. It can be so gradual that maybe not even you will notice. And who knows, maybe their favorite brand will start making their product with more healthy ingredients in the future. Even as we write this book, food manufacturers are changing. I have seen products that have come out with a notice on the front of their package stating "No High Fructose Corn Syrup". Pepsi has come out with a product called "Pepsi Throw Back", containing only sugar for a sweetener. If you are a coke person you can get those glass bottles of Mexican cokes, even in discount grocery stores. One bottle will last 2-3 days because the sugar will make you feel full. Most of the products at the high-end small grocery stores have most of their sweet foods with cane juice or cane sugar. Walmart has a line called Great Value products which use sugar. But, remember, don't start things too fast. That is the mistake everyone makes when they go on a diet or food change plan. They see themselves losing weight and want to hurry it up. You can't do that. Remember the salt story. It took me 6 months to get off salt. Your body has to change back to normal and this means making an entirely new "signal" system in each of your cells. This takes time. If you try this too fast you will not stick to it. Remember that high fructose corn syrup is about 2.3 times sweeter than sucrose so you have to get used to food which is less sweet. And don't try to give up anything else at the same time. It will just frustrate you.

The following is a timeline suggestion for gradual change to achieve a slow weight loss of about 3-4 pounds per month. You do not have to give up anything; just take out the high fructose corn syrup. But, your body will adjust and you should find yourself less hungry and eating less. And remember, exercise is always a good thing.

MONTH#1- FAST FOOD EATING

1. Starting now, purchase only drinks that have no high fructose corn syrup in them.

    That's either at home or out at restaurants. At home, if you are like me you want a carbonated drink with your food. Try carbonated water in a can and add a teaspoon of sugar and lemon or lime juice. Be careful to read the labels because some have been sweetened with high fructose corn syrup. If you prefer, get the Mexican cokes or Pepsi Throwback. At the fast food places, get the water or drink the juice. And, never, ever, get refills. It is not a money saver, it will make you and your kids overweight and sick. You will have to do this slowly because your kids probably love those soft drinks. If your kids drink constantly from those little juice cartons be sure it is a brand without high fructose corn syrup. Now is also the time to delete the artificial sweeteners. Be sure to do this slowly!

2. <u>When you eat out take the list of foods without high fructose corn syrup in them from each of the places.</u>

We have listed them separately in the Appendix so you can take the book or even tear out the page and keep it in your car. Try to order only those foods without the high fructose corn syrup in them. You may have to do that gradually if your kids have a favorite food.

3. <u>If you go to a fancy restaurant try to order plain foods.</u>

Steak is really OK, they don't add high fructose corn syrup to it. Bake potatoes are fine. And restaurants usually use sugar in their desserts. But, avoid stuff with sauces because you won't be able to tell what is in it. If you have a favorite food at your favorite fancy place, lookup the contents online before you go. Decide then what you will do, either change to something else or eat much less of it. If you go without and feel like you have shortchanged yourself...eat a dessert, but, one with sugar and not high fructose corn syrup in it!

4. <u>From now on, when you shop to replace the pre-cooked food, like frozen pizza, buy only from our lists.</u>

We have written a very long list of just frozen pizza, frozen dinners, and many other items which you can substitute for the brands that you already use. And, we did not go to those fancy organic food stores, just the discounts, like you. If necessary, you can add one teaspoon of sugar to a food and then gradually decrease it until the food tastes sweet enough for you.

Promise not to weigh yourself until after one month.

MONTH#2 – YOUR KITCHEN FAST TURNOVERS

1. <u>Replace items with ones from our list.</u>

Buy only cake, biscuit, brownie or corn bread mixes that have no HFCS when you replace items. Any condiments that you run out of this month, for instance catsup, relish, barbeque or other sauces, mayonnaise, syrup, coffee creamers, peanut butter, jelly, juice, salad dressings, or anything else kept in the door of your refrigerator, replace with one on the list, or check labels yourself to avoid HFCS. You do not have to throw things out, just replace them. Buy only cookies, cakes or pies with no HFCS. Replace all baby food with items without high fructose corn syrup, no artificial sweeteners, or food dyes.

2. <u>Take track of how much stuff in your kitchen still has high fructose corn syrup in it.</u>

Now make a decision. Now weigh yourself. If you want to lose weight faster you will have to get rid of it faster.

Month #3 – Replacing the Slow Moving Items

1. <u>Take stock of the pantry and refrigerator.</u>

    There are probably items in the back that came with the house. Check those dates. It really is not good to use outdated items as they may have bacteria in them. Throw those out and replace them with the item without high fructose corn syrup in them. Finish your final and total replacement.

2. <u>Take stock of Yourself and Your Family</u>

    You can probably find some things in their diets to change. How about those foods at school? Can you pack a lunch or become more active in the lunch program? Schools are getting better about the soft drinks and snacks but what about the other food? Send them off with only healthy snacks.

Month#4 – The Replacement Package

1. <u>Buy only fast foods with no HFCS by this time.</u>

    Your body and those of your kids will have adjusted to a less sweet type of food by this time.

2. <u>Buy only dairy products like yogurt, ice cream, whipped cream, margarine, or cheese with no HFCS.</u>

At this time you should also substitute the artificial sweeteners and coffee creamers to either dairy products or items without high fructose corn syrup. Sometimes you may have to just eliminate something. But be sure to do this slowly. I still have not been able to go over to black coffee. I have to add a teaspoon of sugar.

3. Throw out all artificial sweeteners and foods with those weird dyes in them.

   Most places offer a clear alternative. Remember, those tiny babies do not even see color that well yet and the use of a bright red baby drink is only for your sake. Babies are very small so the dose that they receive is much greater than you would get.

4. If possible, Go to Glass or Wax Cartons.

   Remember that all of those BPA's will change the estrogen levels in your blood and further cause you and your family to gain weight. Never microwave anything in its plastic container. Remove it and put it on a glass plate or bowl first. If you must use plastic baby bottles use the ones with those rolls of plastic inserts and be sure not to microwave or heat them. Heat the formula in a glass container then pour into the plastic insert. And only use that insert once.

By the end of four months you should be totally aware of what you are buying and eating and everyone else in your family will be aware too. Some of you will have dropped a few pounds if you were overweight. From the experience of those in my class the weight loss varies from 2-5 pounds per month. They eat mostly fast foods so you may be able to control this more.

But always remember, this is not a quick diet. It is a change in lifestyle. We believe that by now, after reading this book, you realize that the obesity trend in this country is mainly due to the food additives that we have ingested. They have tricked our metabolism into changing patterns toward fat accumulation and have made us constantly hungry. This was originally not your fault. But now that you know this you must act.

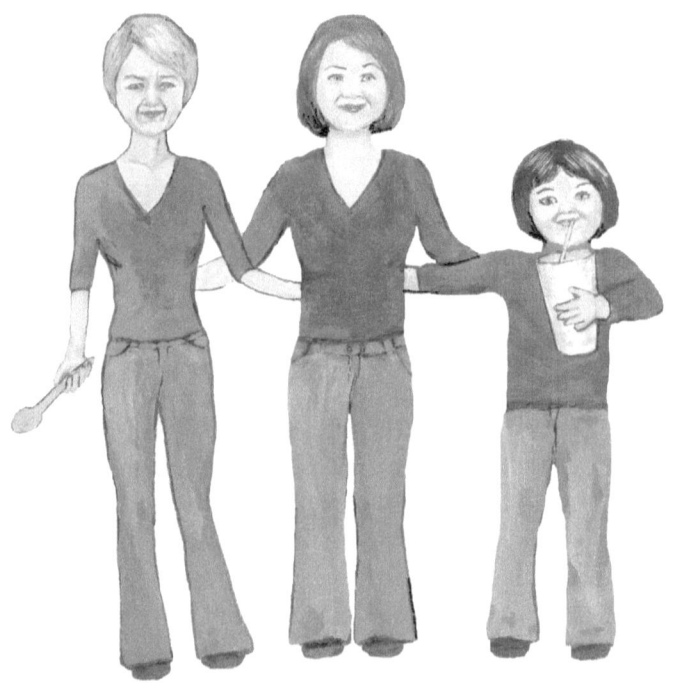

We know that you want to be healthy and give your children the best chance at a long and healthy life. It is always hard to start a new good habit. But when you see results it encourages you to keep up the good work. Many of my students had been overweight or obese for most of their lives. Some already had pre-diabetes. Many have changed their trends. We hope you try these simple steps. You'll all feel better, look better and improve your chances of a long, successful and healthy life.

APPENDIX

Products that do NOT contain High Fructose Corn Syrup*

Baking and Cooking Ingredients
- Betty Crocker 7-Layer Bar(mix)
- Betty Crocker Dark Chocolate Brownie mix
- Betty Crocker cake icing
- Betty Crocker Bisquick
- Betty Crocker cake mix
- Pillsbury Frosting
- Betty Crocker pie crust
- Nestle condensed milk

Beverages
- Northland Cranberry Juice
- Abbott Laboratories Pedia Sure
- China/Mexico Cola
- Dr.Pepper (original formula)
- Pepsi Throwback
- Jones Soda (recently announced that they were going back to real sugar)
- Goose Island soda (Root Beer, Orange Soda)
- Calistoga Juice Squeeze
- Carnation Instant Breakfast
- Simply Orange juice products
- Simply Lemonade
- Silk soy milk
- Tropicana OJ

- Minute Maid Orange Juice
- Monster energy drinks
- Swiss Miss cocoa mix
- Nestle Coffee Mate creamers
- Nestle NesQuik Chocolate Milk Mix
- Nestle NesQuik Chocolate Milk (bottled)
- Nestle "Abuelita" Chocolate Syrup (Hispanic Section)
- R.W. Knudsen Recharge (sports drink)
- Starbuck's frappuccinos (bottled)
- Fuze Drinks
- TeaZazz
- Vivi Smart Soda
- Gatorade
- Kool-Aid
- Capri Sun
- Nestle Juicy Juice
- Ocean Spray juices
- V8 juice

Bread
- Pepperidge Farms whole grain honey oat
- Nature's Own Sugar Free 100% Whole Grain bread
- Nature's Own -Honey 7 Grain
- Nature's Own 100% whole wheat
- Martins Potato breads and rolls
- Thomas's Low Carb English Muffins
- Thomas Hearty Grain Honey Wheat English Muffins
- Best Choice English Muffins
- Nature's Own -Healthline Sugar Free Whole wheat
- Ezekiel 4:9 sprouted grain breads (in freezer section)
- Francisco International *Extra* Sour Dough bread (the regular Sour Dough has it!)
- Pepperidge Farm Honey Wheatberry

- Milton's Wheat and Multi-grain bread
- Bagels from a local Jewish bakery
- Kirkland brand (Costco) multigrain bread
- Sara Lee Cinnamon Raisin
- Sara Lee 100% Whole Wheat bread
- Pepperidge Farm whole grain bagel
- Thomas's plain bagels
- Matthew's All Natural Bread
- Amana Multi Grain Bread
- Country Hearth 12-Grain Bread
- Earth Grains 100% Natural 7-Grain Bread
- Orrow Wheat Bread – most varieties
- Rays New York Bagels
- Whole Foods store brand hot dog and hamburger buns (they are whole wheat)
- FlatOut Bread
- Alternative Bagel --- sweat wheat
- Pillsbury crescent rolls
- Pillsbury biscuits

Breakfast Cereals
- Post Grape-Nuts
- Quaker Oats Life Cereal/Cinnamon Life
- Quaker Oatmeal
- Quaker Instant Oatmeal
- General Mills Cheerios
- Most cereals labeled "Organic"
- Kashi Go Lean (original and Crunch)
- Kellogg's Honey Smacks
- Kellogg's Corn Pops
- Barabara's Puffins
- Chex Cereals (Wheat, Rice and Corn)
- Kroger Apple Dapples
- Great Value fruit and cream instant oatmeal
- Post Waffle Crisp
- Post Fruity Pebbles

- Mom's Best Natural Cereals (all varieties)

Breakfast Pastries / Waffles / Granola Bars
- Eggo Nutrigrain Blueberry
- Kashi Go Lean and Heart to Heart Waffles
- The TLC granola bars, by Kashi, all are HFCS free
- Sunbelt cereal bars
- Nature Valley Roasted Nut Crunch bars
- Kashi Bars
- Odwalla Bars
- Quaker Chewy Granola Bars

Candy and Other Sweets
- Lindt Lindor truffles (balls)
- Cost Plus World Market has a lot of imported candy from Germany that I've found to be HFCS free.
- Kellogg's Yogos Bits
- Hostess Donettes
- Little Debbie Peanut Butter Crunch bars
- Little Debbie Swiss Rolls
- Little Debbie Chocolate Chip Cream Pies
- Cloverhill donuts
- Jello Mousse pudding
- Sugar free Jello
- Betty Crocker Fruit Roll Ups
- Welch's Fruit Snacks
- Jolly Rancher hard candy
- Twizzlers
- Skittles
- Jello pudding
- Kraft Marshmallows
- Hunt's Snack Pack tapioca pudding

Condiments
- Heinz organic tomato ketchup
- Hunt's ketchup

- French's Worcestershire
- Tartar Sauce, most varieties
- Farman's pickle relish
- Mt. Olive Hamburger dill chips
- Annie's Natural Organic Ketchup
- Frenchs Honey Dijon Mustard (I don't think most regular mustard contains hfcs, but a lot of the "honey" mustard does, which is why I'm listing some honey mustards here that don't.)
- Woeber Sweet And Spicy Mustard
- Consorzio Bbq Sauce Organic Original
- Whole Foods 365 Ketchup (both regular and Organic)
- Kroger cocktail sauce

Cookies and Cakes
- Pepperidge Farm Chessmen cookies -- plain and the new chocolate
- Kedem Tea Biscuits (reg. and chocolate) --- found in the Kosher section
- Paul Newman sandwich cookies
- Kashi line of cookies
- Back to Nature peanut butter sandwich cookies
- Destrooper Almond Thins Cookie
- Destrooper Butter Crisp Cookies
- Keebler Pecan Sandies Cookies
- Keebler Simply Sandies Cookies
- Lu Le Petit Beurre Cookies
- Lu Scottish Recipe Shortbread
- Mi-Del Snaps Ginger
- Newmans Wheat Free Fig Newton Cookies
- Newmans Own Ginger Os Ginger N Creme Cookies
- NewmanS Own Alphabet Cookies
- Pepperidge Farms Butter Chessman Cookies
- Pepperidge Farm 100% Natural Varieties
- Nestle Tolls House cookie dough

Chocolate
- Cadbury - Most Varieties
- Hershey's Symphony
- Hershey's 100 Calorie Wafer Bar
- Hershey Skor Candy Bar
- Hershey Special Dark Candy Bar
- Hershey Kisses
- Dove - Most varieties
- Reeses Peanut Butter Cups
- Most Imported (Europe) and Organic chocolate
- M&M's
- Toll House chocolate chips

Crackers
- Annies - Cheddar cheese bunnies and honey graham bunnies
- Wasa Crisp Breads (all varieties)
- Atheno's baked pita chips
- Stacey's Naked Pita bread chips *note, have not seen HFCS in Hummus
- Dare Vinta Crackers
- Nabisco Triscuits
- Great Value (Walmart's brand) cracked wheat rounds
- Stone Ground (the white square crackers from Canada)

Dairy
- Brown Cow vanilla yogurt
- Southern Home Nonfat Plain Yogurt
- Dannon Plain Yogurt
- Mountain High Yogurt (it *appears* all varieties are HFCS free)
- Dannon All Natural Vanilla Yogurt
- Dannon All Natural Coffee Yogurt
- Dannon Greek Yogurt (any)

- Dannon Activia Yogurt
- Yoplait Gogurt Yogurt
- Horizon Organic Fat Free Yogurt
- Nancys Reduced Fat Plain
- Nancy's Whole Milk Honey Yogurt
- Stoneyfield Farm Yobaby Yogurt

Fruits and Vegetables - Canned and Dried
- Motts Natural (No Sugar Added)Apple Sauce
- Most no sugar added packed fruit --- please check labels
- Bush's baked beans
- Del Monte sliced peaches
- Del Monte fruit cups
- Sunsweet Prunes
- Ocean Spray dried cranberries

Ice Cream
- Breyers - All Natural Coffee
- Breyers - All Natural Cherry Vanilla
- Breyers - All Natural Mint Chocolate Chip
- Luigi Italian Ice
- Blue Bunny All Natural Vanilla
- Blue Bunny sherbert

Jam, Jelly, Syrup, Spreads
- Skippy Peanut Butter
- Smuckers Jif Peanut Butter
- Smuckers Peanut Butter
- Costco makes an organic peanut butter
- Whole Foods brand peanut butter
- Blue Bonnet margarine
- Kraft Philadelphia Cream Cheese
- Best Choice light syrup
- Karo Dark (with Blue label)
- Karo Brown Sugar syrup

- Hero Jams (from Swizterland) --- can be found at Cost Plus World Market
- Darbo Jams (from Austria) --- can be found at Cost Plus World Market
- Whole foods brand (365) strawberry jam
- Sarabeth Jam
- Smuckers organic grape jelly
- Safeway "O" Organics Maple Syrup
- Harry and David Ancho sweet chili pepper spread

Pastries
- Try your local, family operated, pastry shop. Since HFCS is added to extend shelf life it is not generally found in family operated bakeries.

Prepared Foods
- Ore-Ida French Fries
- Nestle Hot Pockets
- Nestle Lean Pockets
- Totinos Pizza Rolls
- DiGiorno Pizza
- Best Choice frozen burritos
- Stouffer's lasagna
- Oscar Mayer Lunchables
- Lunchmeat, most brands
- Gerber baby food
- Betty Crocker boxed potatoes
- Hormel Spam
- Rice A Roni
- Ramen noodles
- Amy's Organic Meals
- Kraft Macaroni and Cheese
- Betty Crocker Hamburger Helper

Salad Dressings
- Great Value (WalMart) Zesty Italian Dressing

- Hellmann's Real Mayonnaise
- Kraft Mayonnaise
- Hidden Valley Ranch Old Fash. Buttermilk
- Blue Plate Mayonnaise
- Ken's Sweet Vidalia Onion dressing
- Annie's Naturals organic papaya poppyseed salad dressing.
- Annie's Naturals Goddess Dressing (check other Annie's too, quite a few are HFCS free)
- Brianna's Homemade Blush Vinaigrette Salad Dressing (all varieties seem to be HFCS free)
- Drew's Salad Dressings
- Most Neumann's varieties
- Kraft Honey Dijon Vinaigrette, dressing & marinade
- Kraft Balsamic Vinaigrette, dressing & marinade
- Kraft Thousand Island Dressing

Sauces
- Barilla Pesto
- Ken's Steak House Honey Teriyaki Marinade
- Kikkoman Soy Sauce
- Soy Vey Very Very Teriyaki --- check marinade section, also Kosher section
- Bullseye BBQ sauce Original
- Ragu pizza sauce
- Ragu tomato sauce
- Pace Salsa

Snacks
- Frito's corn chips
- Natural Cheetos
- Lay's Honey BBQ chips
- General Mills Chex Mix
- Quaker Rice Cakes
- Jack Link's Beef Jerky

- Popcorn, most varieties
- Planter's Peanuts

Soups
- Annie's Organic Soups

* This list is not meant to be all-inclusive. If your product was not listed here please inform us and we can include it on our website.

Caloric Intake Assignment

Biochemistry Assignment for Biochemistry and Society

Caloric Intake

Below are listed the recommended caloric intake for students in my class. This list is for moderately active individuals. Individuals who are more active can add an extra 500 calories.

Caloric intake for moderately-active males: 10 to 24 Years of Age: 3,000 calories/day

Caloric intake for moderately-active females: 19 to 34 Years of Age: 2,100 calories/day

A. Using these values and the USDA nutritional guide (see website listed below) calculate the # of calories you ingest <u>over 3 days</u>. All meals and snacks should be counted. You may have to guess at your portion sizes. Be sure to count the calories in the beverages you drink as well. <u>Show all work</u>. If you need to convert oz to calories use 4 cal for each gram of carbs or protein and 9 cal for fats and oils.

Great resources can be found at the following sites:
http://www.mypyramidtracker.gov
http://www.nutritiondata.com

B. Calculate the daily % of calories you had from fat, from carbohydrates and from proteins.

C. Make a list of what you are deficient in and how you could improve your own daily diet.

D. List how many calories and per cent are from carbohydrates.

E. List how many of your foods contained high fructose corn syrup.

INGREDIENTS ASSIGNMENT

Biochemistry Assignment for Biochemistry and Society

Identify the food item based on the list of ingredients taken from the product packaging.

See list below.

1. _____Sorbitol, water, hydrated silica, PEG-32, sodium lauryl sulfate, SDalcohol 38-B, flavor, cellulose gum, sodium saccharin, titanium dioxide, sodium, monofluorophosphate

2. _____Water, cetyl alcohol, tocopheryl acetate, honeysuckle extract, aloevera gel, Cetrimonium chloride, disodium EDTA, DMDM hydantoin, methylchloroisothiazolidine, propylene glycol, methylisothiazolinone, FD&C dyes yellow #5 and Blue #1.

3. _____Dicalcium phosphate, Sorbitol, Magnesium phosphate, sodiumascorbate, gelatin, Ferrous fumarate, flavors, starch, Stearic acid, tocopheryl acetate, carrageenan, magnesium strearate, niacinamide, zinc oxide, hydrogenated vegetable oil, calcium pantothenate, FD&C dyes Red #40, Blue #2, Yellow #6, aspartame, cupricoxide, pyridoxine hydrochloride, trans-retinol, riboflavin, thiamine mononitrate, Monoammonium glycyrrhizinate, beta carotene, folic acid, potassium iodide, cholecalciferol, biotin, magnesium oxide, cobalalmine.

4. _____Stock, modified corn starch, salt, wheat flour, monosodium glutamate, animal fat, partially hydrogenated vegetable oils (canola, cottonseed and soy), whey, autolyzed yeast extract, sodium caseinate, soy protein isolate, maltodextrin, spice, mono and diglycerides, mono and dipotassium phosphate, natural flavor, tumeric, caramelcoloring, soy lecithin.

5. _____Wheat flour, wheat bran, beef meal, bone meal, milk, wheat germ, animal fat, salt, dicalcium phosphate, calcium carbonate, zinc sulfate, copper sulfate, ethylenediamine dihydriodide, brewer's yeast, malted barley flour, poultry digest, dried cheese, sodium metabisulfite, choline chloride, D,L-alpha tocopheryl acetate, trans-retinol acetate, calcium pantothenate, riboflavin, cobalamine, D-activated animal sterol, natural flavor

6. _____Carbonated water, high fructose corn syrup and/or sugar, concentrated orange juice and other natural flavors, citric acid, sodium benzoate, caffeine, sodium citrate, gum arabic, erythorbic acid, calcium disodium EDTA and brominated vegetable oil, yellow dye #5

Shampoo, gravy, vitamin supplement, hair conditioner, Milk Bones, instant soup, toothpaste, granola bar, prepared pudding, tofu, Mountain Dew®.

7. Now see if you can find out what each is, using the internet or FDA site online.

Label Assignment

Biochemistry Assignment for Biochemistry and Society

1. Find and include the label with the project. It must have at least 20 listed ingredients. Make it something that you eat regularly.

2. List each ingredient and give the group that it belongs to – lipid, carbohydrate, nucleotide or protein/amino acid. Give the chemical and common name. Draw out the chemical structure for 5 of these ingredients. You will not get credit for the formula. You must draw out the entire structure. You can find them on Wikipedia.

3. Now separately list each of the ingredients which have no nutritional value (an example would be yellow dye 2) and define their purpose.

4. Sometimes it will list "flavors added", so assume they have no nutritional value but see if you can guess what they are.

5. List the percentages of daily calories, carbohydrates, and fats that one serving contains. List the percent trans fats. This will be under Nutritional Information, not under ingredients.

6. List all of the ingredients that have nutritional value. Name three other sources of these nutrients (not the compound but the nutrient). For example, casein is in milk but it is a protein...where else can you get protein?

7. Select 3 ingredients and describe which organ metabolizes each, and, how they are used in fat cells, liver, brain and/or muscle. See the FDA site online.

www.fda.gov/food/labelingnutrition/
consumerinformation/ucm078889.htm

8. How much salt is present in the food item? What percent of the recommended daily allowance (RDA) does that amount represent?

9. Identify potential health risks associated with three of the ingredients with regard to its presence in the food or the amount present. This could be, as an example, trans fats, or saturated vs unsaturated fats or cholesterol.

10. Is high fructose corn syrup in your food? It may also be listed as fructose corn syrup, corn syrup, or even corn sygar.

References

READ THE LABEL

1. Yang, C., Yaniger, S., Jordan, C., Klein, D., and Bittner, G. (2011) Most Plastic Products Release Estrogenic Chemicals: A Potential Health Problem that Can be Solved. Environmental Health Perspectives. Online ,doi:10.1289/ehp.1003220, http://dx.doi.org/

2. Phthalate – http://en.wikipedia.org/wiki/Phthalate

3. Newbold, R. (2010) Impact of environmental endocrine disrupting chemicals on the development of obesity. Hormones, 9:206-217.

4. Desvergne, B., Feige, J., Casals-Casas, C. (2009) PPAR-mediated activity of phthalates: A link to the obesity epidemic? Molecular and Cellular Endocrinology. 304: 43-48.

5. Kim, B., Cho, S., Kim, Y., et al. (2009) Phthalates exposure and attention-deficit/hyperactivity disorder in school-age children. Biol. Psychiatry. 66:958-963.

6. Sax, L. (2010) Polyethylene Terephthalate may yield endocrine disruptors. Environmental Health Perspectives. 118:445-448.

DOES YOUR BODY KNOW THE DIFFERENCE -

1. http://www.netmums.com/food/Food_NastiesWatch_Out_.321/

2. http://en.wikipedia.org/wiki/High-fructose_corn_syrup

3. http://foodproductdesign.com/articles/2008/12hfcs-how-sweet-it-is. aspx

4. http://www.agr.gc.ca/AAFC-AAC/display-afficher. do?id=1172167862291&lang=eng

5. Hanover, L.M., White, J.S. 1993. Manufacturing composition, and applications of fructose. Am. J. Clin Nutri. 58 (suppl):724S-732S.

6. http://www.SweetSurprise.com

7. http://www.foodnavigator-usa.com/Financial-Industry/CRA-petitions-FDA-for-high-fructose; http://well.blogs.nytimes.com/2010/14/a-new-name-for-high-fructose-corn-syrup/

8. Tappy, L. and Le, K. (2010) Metabolic Effects of Fructose and the Worldwide Increase in Obesity. Physiol. Rev 90:23-46.

9. Marshal, R., and Kooi, E. (1957) Enzymatic conversion of D-glucose to D-fructose. Sciences. 125(3249) 648-649.

10. Yakasaki, Y. Patent: Inventor, Agency of Industrial Science and Technology, Japan. Patent Title: Enzymatic Method for Manufacture of Fructose from Glucose; Application Number:05/083/168, Filed Oct 23, 1970.

11. Lindemann, B. (2001) Receptors and Transduction in Taste. Nature. 413:194-202.

12. Narishima, R., Yamasaki, M., Hasegawa, S., Yoshida, S., Tanaka, S., Fukui, T.(2010) Leptin controls ketone body utilization in hypothalamic neuron. Neuroscience. Letters. Dor:10.1016/j.neulet.2010.11.081.

13. Havel, P. (1997) Glucose but not fructose infusion increases circulating leptin in proportion to adipose stores in rhesus monkeys. Exp. Clin. Endocrinol. Diabetes. 105:37-38.

14. Schwartz, M., Woods, S., Porte, D., Seeley, R., Baskin, D. (2000) Central nervous system control of food intake. Nature. 404: 661-670.

15. Huang, W., Dedousis, N., Bhatt, B., O'Doherty, R. (2004) Impaired activation of phosphatidylinositol 3-kinase by leptin is a novel mechanism of hepatic resistance in diet-induced obesity. J. Biol. Chem. 279:21695-21700.

16. Erickson, J. Hollopeter, G., Palmiter, R. (1996) Attenuation of the obesity syndrome of *ob/ob* mice by the loss of neuropeptide Y. Science. 274:1704-1707.

17. Lucinio, J., et al. (2004) Phenotypic effects of leptin replacement on morbid obesity, diabetes mellitus, hypogonadism, and behavior in leptin-deficient adults. Proc. Natl. Acad. Sci. U.S.A. 101:4531-4536.

18. Teff, K., et al. (2004) Dietary fructose reduces circulating insulin and leptin, attenuates postprandial suppression of ghrelin, and increases triglycerides in women. J. Clin. Endocrinol.& Metab. 89(6): 2963-2972.

19. Swarbrick, M., et al. (2008) Consumption of fructose-sweetened beverages for 10 weeks increases postprandial triacylglycerol and apolipoprotein-B concentrations in overweight and obese women. British J. of Nutrition. 100:947-952.

20. Bocarsly, M., Powell, E., Avena, N., Hoebel, B. (2010) High-fructose corn syrup causes characteristics of obesity in rats: Increased body weight, body fat, and triglyceride levels. Pharmacol. Biochemistry, and Behavior. 97:101-106.

21. http://en.wikipedia.org/wiki/Leptin.

22. http://en.wikipedia.org/wiki/Neuropeptide_Y.

23. http://en.wikipedia.org/wiki/Ghrelin.

24. http://en.wikipedia.org/wiki/Peptide_YY.

25. Yang, Q. (2010) Gain weight by "going diet?" Artificial sweeteners and the neurobiology of sugar cravings. Yale Journal of Biology and Medicine. 83:101-108.

26. Humphries, P., Pretorius, E., and Naude, H. (2008) Direct and indirect cellular effects of aspartame on the brain. European Journal of Clinical Nutrition. 62:451-462.

27. Ciappuccini, R., Anselmant, T., Maillefert, J., Tavernier, C., and Ornetti, P. (2010) Aspartame-induced fibromyalgia, an unusual btu curable cause of chronic pain. Clin. Exp. Rheumatol. 6 Suppl 63:S131-3.

METABOLIC SYNDROME

1. Ervin, R. (2009) Prevalence of Metabolic Syndrome Among Adults 20 Years of age and Over, by Sex, Age, Race, and Ethnicity, and Body Mass Index: United States, 2003-2006. National Health Statistics Reports. Number 13, May 5, 2009. US, HHS.

2. http://healthhubs.net/heartdisease/waist-size-predicts-heart-disease-risk-better-than-bmi/

3. http://en.wikipedia.org/wiki/C-reactive_protein

4. Huang, D., Dhawan, T., Young, S., et al. (2011) Fructose impairs glucose-induced hepatic triglyceride synthesis. Lipids In Health and Disease. 10:1-10.

5. Stanhope, K., and Havel, P. (2010) Fructose consumption: Recent results and their potential implications. Annals of the New York Academy of Sciences. 1190:15-24.

6. Stanhope, K., and Havel, P. (2008) Endocrine and metabolic effects of consuming beverages sweetened with fructose, glucose, sucrose, or high-fructose corn syrup. Am. J. Clin. Nutr. 88(suppl): 1733S-1737S.

7. Soleimani, M. (2010) Dietary fructose, salt absorption and hypertension in metabolic syndrome: towards a new paradigm. (2011) Acta Physiol. 201:55-62.

8. Stanhope, K., Schwarz, J., Keim, N., et al. (2009) Consuming fructose-sweetened, not glucose-sweetened, beverages increases visceral adiposity and lipids and decreases insulin sensitivity in overweight/obese humans. J. Clin. Invest. 119:1322-1334.

9. Rizkalla, S. (2010) Health implications of fructose consumption: A review of recent data. Nutrition and Metabolism. 7:82-99.

About The Authors

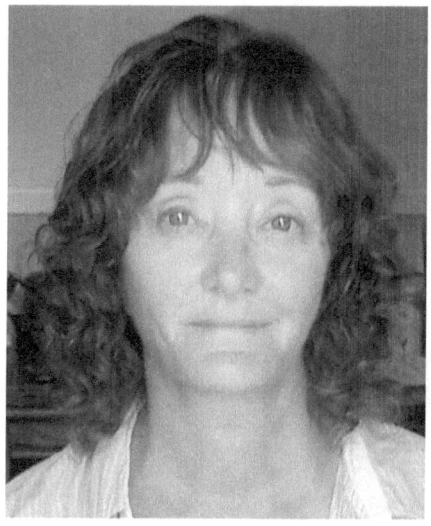

Dr. Dee Takemoto is a Professor of Biochemistry at Kansas State University, in Manhattan, KS, for 32 years. She teaches currently to non-science majors, especially to emphasize the knowledge of health issues. She has recently co-authored a textbook and lab manual, "Molecules and Society", which is now in a beta edition to students (published by Kendall Hunt). Dr. Takemoto has had a long-standing interest in diets and health and has been quoted, internationally, on the BBC for her work with anti-oxidants in wheat. She has published over 100 scientific papers and holds research grants from the National Eye Institute of the National Institutes of Health. The current book grew from her lectures to students who had a desire to be healthy and lose weight. Dr. Takemoto resides in Manhattan, KS, during the school year, and, in her home in Aptos, California when school is not in session.

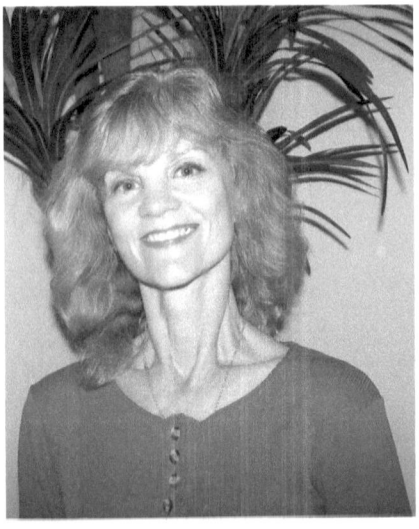

Joanne McIntyre is a practicing echocardiographer in a pediatric cardiology practice in Pasadena, Ca. She has a lifetime interest in health and diet issues. Throughout her career, she has observed children who struggled with weight and health issues. She is an artist, writer, and she resides in Sierra Madre, California. Joanne and Dee are sisters.